Mechanics of Sport

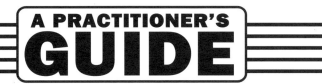

A PRACTITIONER'S GUIDE

Gerry Carr

University of Victoria

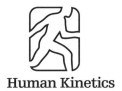

Human Kinetics

Library of Congress Cataloging-in-Publication Data

Carr, Gerald A., 1936-
    Mechanics of sport : a practitioner's guide / Gerry Carr.
      p. cm.
    Includes bibliographical references and index.
    ISBN 0-87322-974-6
    1. Kinesiology. 2. Human mechanics. 3. Sports--Physiological
aspects.   I. Title.
QP303.C375   1997
612'.044--dc20

95-52859
CIP

ISBN: 0-87322-974-6

Developmental Editor: Marni Basic; **Assistant Editors**: Susan Moore-Kruse, John Wentworth, and Dawn Cassady; **Editorial Assistants**: Amy Carnes and Jennifer J. Hemphill; **Copyeditors**: Denelle Eknes and Anne Mischakoff Heiles; **Proofreader**: Jim Burns; **Indexer**: Theresa J. Schaefer; **Graphic Artist**: Angela K. Snyder; **Graphic Designer**: Robert Reuther; **Photo Editor**: Boyd LaFoon, **Cover Designer**: Jack Davis; **Photographer (cover)**: Dave Black; **Illustrator**: Paul To; **Mac Artist**: Craig Ronto; **Printer**: Versa Press

Printed in the United States of America   10 9 8 7 6 5 4 3 2

Human Kinetics
Web site: http://www.humankinetics.com/

United States: Human Kinetics
P.O. Box 5076
Champaign, IL 61825-5076
1-800-747-4457
e-mail: humank@hkusa.com

Canada: Human Kinetics, Box 24040,
Windsor, ON N8Y 4Y9
1-800-465-7301 (in Canada only)
e-mail: humank@hkcanada.com

Europe: Human Kinetics
P.O. Box IW14, Leeds LS16 6TR, United Kingdom
(44) 1132 781708
e-mail: humank@hkeurope.com

Australia: Human Kinetics, 57A Price Avenue
Lower Mitcham, South Australia 5062
(08) 277 1555
e-mail: humank@hkaustralia.com

New Zealand: Human Kinetics, P.O. Box 105-231,
Auckland 1
(09) 523 3462
e-mail: humank@hknewz.com

To all who want to understand how superior sport techniques
are based on the best use of scientific concepts and natural laws.

CONTENTS

FOREWORD

Outstanding athletic performances require a timely meld of many factors. They require an appropriate physique, excellent physical conditioning, and the psychological attributes necessary to bring everything together at the right time. They also require an appropriate technique (appropriate ways of moving the head, trunk, and limbs). It is this effective technique, and the science of mechanics underlying it, that is the focus of Gerry Carr's book.

The importance of a knowledge of mechanics to an understanding of techniques in sport, dance, rehabilitation, and, indeed, all human movement, has long been recognized. Teachers, coaches, clinicians, and performers are seriously handicapped if they lack knowledge of the mechanics that form the underpinning of the techniques they teach and use. They are at a disadvantage when it comes to such matters as selecting the best technique to use, deciding how to modify a particular technique to allow for the personal characteristics of the performer, observing faults and identifying their causes, and devising ways to correct these faults.

The science of mechanics is traditionally taught with frequent reference to the algebra, trigonometry, calculus, and other branches of mathematics from which it derives. This obviously presents a formidable barrier to those who are not already well-versed in basic mathematics. Teachers of the mechanics of human movement have often sought to overcome this obstacle by simplifying the mathematical treatment and, where possible, presenting the basic concepts in nonmathematical terms. Gerry Carr has boldly taken this process one step farther. He has eliminated formal mathematical treatment entirely. There are no formulas or calculations in *Mechanics of Sport*.

This is a book for coaches, teachers, athletes, and sport fans, presented in simple, nonmathematical terms and containing a host of interesting, practical examples drawn from the literature and from Gerry's own extensive background in athletics. It is a book that is easy to read and one that promises to make an understanding of mechanics and sport available to a much wider audience than has been reached by previous texts in this field.

James G. Hay, PhD
University of Iowa

ACKNOWLEDGMENTS

I very much appreciate the assistance from Larry Yore, Jim Haddow, Keith Russell, and James Hay, and the encouragement and continued support from the members of the faculty of the School of Physical Education, University of Victoria, British Columbia, Canada. I also want to thank the enthusiastic and supportive students in the sport mechanics classes at the University of Victoria—the guinea pigs for the testing of my explanations of the principles discussed in this text. Lastly, I want to thank my wife, Catherine, who by now knows this text as well as I do!

CREDITS

Figure 2.6b: Adapted, by permission, from G. Dyson, 1986, *Mechanics of athletics*, 8th ed. (London: Hodder & Stoughton Educational).

Figure 2.12:   Reprinted, by permission, from S.J. Hall, 1995, *Basic biomechanics*, 2nd ed. (St. Louis: Mosby-Year Book, Inc.), 313.

Figure 2.13:   From E. Kreighbaum and K.M. Barthels, *Biomechanics: A qualitative approach for studying human movement*. Copyright © 1990. All rights reserved. Adapted by permission of Allyn & Bacon.

Figure 3.7:   Adapted, by permission, from S.L. Blanding and J.M. Monteleone, 1992, *What makes a boomerang come back: The science of sports* (Stamford, CT: Longmeadow).

Figure 3.9a, b, and c: From *The tour de France complete book of cycling* by David Chavner & Michael Halstead. Copyright © 1990 by David Chavner & Michael Halstead. Reprinted by permission of Random House, Inc.

Figure 4.18:   From Kathryn Luttgens, et al., *Kinesiology: Scientific basis of human motion*, 8th edition. Copyright © 1992. Wm. C. Brown Communications, Inc. Reprinted by permission of Times Mirror Higher Education Group, Inc., Dubuque, Iowa. All rights reserved.

Figure 4.21a and b: Adapted, with permission, from H. Braecklin, 1974, *Trampolinturnen II* (Germany: Limpert Verlag), 29.

Figure 4.41a and b: From Marlene J. Adrian and John M. Cooper, *Biomechanics of human movement*, 2nd edition. Copyright © 1995. Wm. C. Brown Communications, Inc. Reprinted by permission of Times Mirror Higher Education Group, Inc., Dubuque, Iowa. All rights reserved.

Figure 4.43:   Adapted, by permission, from G. Rackham, 1975, *Diving complete* (London: Faber & Faber Ltd.).

Figure 6.3:   From Kathryn Luttgens, et al., *Kinesiology: Scientific basis of human motion*, 8th edition. Copyright © 1992. Wm. C. Brown Communications, Inc. Reprinted by permission of Times Mirror Higher Education Group, Inc., Dubuque, Iowa. All rights reserved.

Figure 6.17:   From J.G. Hay and J.G. Reid, *Anatomy, mechanics, and human motion*, 2nd ed. Copyright © 1988. All rights reserved. Adapted by permission of Allyn & Bacon.

Figure 6.18a and b: Adapted from *Swimming faster* by Ernest Maglischo by permission of Mayfield Publishing Company. Copyright © 1983 by Mayfield Publishing Company.

Figure 6.20a and b: From E. Kreighbaum and K.M. Barthels, *Biomechanics: A aualitative approach for studying human movement*. Copyright © 1990. All rights reserved. Adapted by permission of Allyn & Bacon.

Figure 6.21:   From E. Kreighbaum and K.M. Barthels, *Biomechanics: A qualitative approach for studying human movement*. Copyright © 1990. All rights reserved. Adapted by permission of Allyn & Bacon.

Figure 6.28:   Reprinted, by permission, from S.J. Hall, 1995, *Basic biomechanics*, 2nd ed. (St. Louis: Mosby-Year Book, Inc.), 487.

Figure 8.1:   From J.G. Hay and J.G. Reid, *Anatomy, mechanics, and human motion*, 2nd ed. Copyright © 1988. All rights reserved. Adapted by permission of Allyn & Bacon.

Figure 8.4:   Adapted from *Swimming faster* by Ernest Maglischo by permission of Mayfield Publishing Company. Copyright © 1983 by Mayfield Publishing Company.

Figure 9.8   From Marlene J. Adrian and John M. Cooper, *Biomechanics of human movement*, 2nd edition. Copyright © 1995. Wm. C. Brown Communications, Inc. Reprinted by permission of Times Mirror Higher Education Group, Inc., Dubuque, Iowa. All rights reserved.

PART ONE

Understanding Mechanics and Sport Technique

CHAPTER 1

Introduction: Making a Smart Move

When you finish reading this chapter, you should be able to explain

- why it's important to have a basic understanding of sport mechanics;

- how knowing sport mechanics can help you teach efficient technique and correct errors in performance;

- how an understanding of sport mechanics can help eliminate a trial and error approach to coaching;

- how a better knowledge of sport mechanics can help athletes improve their techniques; and

- how a knowledge of sport mechanics can help in assessing the value of sport equipment and new ways of performing sport skills.

Mechanics of Sport has been written for coaches, teachers, athletes, and sport fans. It tells you how a knowledge of sport mechanics helps to produce better performances. Those of you who coach will find that *Mechanics of Sport* helps you become a better coach. Those of you who are athletes will discover that the information in *Mechanics of Sport* helps improve your performances. *Mechanics of Sport* is even valuable to those of you who neither coach nor compete but who are enthusiastic sport fans. You'll find that *Mechanics of Sport* helps you become more critical and appreciative observers of the sports you love.

When you read *Mechanics of Sport* you'll find that it doesn't concentrate on any particular sport—like football, rowing, or basketball—or on any specific sport skill—like punting, passing, serving, or spiking. Instead, *Mechanics of Sport* explains how and why a basic understanding of mechanical principles helps produce an improved performance. If you're coaching, you'll be able to look at an athlete's performance and say to yourself, "Some of the actions in the athlete's technique are good. But there are actions that are inefficient and need correcting. What I know of mechanics tells me that they're wrong, and I know what kind of movements should replace them. When the corrections are made, the athlete will have a more efficient technique and produce a better performance."

Sport Mechanics

Scientists who work in the field of mechanics study the effects of forces (like gravity, friction, and air resistance) on living and nonliving objects. They use their knowledge of mechanics to help design objects that we use in everyday life, such as buildings, bridges, automobiles, boats, and planes. In addition, they assess the effect of forces on humans and, vice versa, the effect of forces applied by humans.

It's obvious that gravity, friction, and air resistance make no distinction between nonsporting and sporting activities! A high jumper fights against gravity just as a person climbing stairs or a plane taking off. Likewise, air resistance and friction oppose both an automobile and an Olympic sprint cyclist. This indicates that the same mechanical principles that are used in our everyday world can also be applied to sport.

Mechanical Principles

In sport, mechanical principles are nothing more than basic rules that govern an athlete's actions. For example, if a coach and an athlete understand the characteristics of the earth's gravitational force, they know what must be done to counteract the effect of this force and, conversely, what actions must be performed to make use of it. A springboard diver who is aware that gravity acts perpendicularly to the earth's surface has a better understanding of what trajectory gives an optimal flight path for a dive. Similarly, wrestlers will learn that gravity is their friend when they've got their opponent off balance. On the other hand, if they don't maintain their own stability, gravity switches sides and teams up with their opponent! Ski jumpers understand that if they flex their legs and bend forward as they slide down the ramp, they reduce air resistance. This body position allows gravity to accelerate them in preparation for the takeoff. Once in flight the ski jumpers counteract the force of gravity by making use of air resistance. They extend their legs and lean forward so that they simulate the wing of a plane. In this way air resistance provides an upward lift force. It is this variation in the use of gravity and air resistance that helps give ski jumpers their long soaring jumps.

There are many more forces on earth besides gravity, air resistance, and friction. These forces act in different ways, and if you're in a contact sport you must also consider the forces produced by your opponents. If you coach and you understand how all these forces interrelate, you are better able to analyze an athlete's technique and improve the athlete's performance. If you are an athlete and you have this knowledge, you'll understand why it's better to apply muscular force at one instant than at another and why movements in your technique are best performed in one manner rather than another. Even as a spectator, you'll find that an understanding of basic mechanical principles helps you become more knowledgeable and appreciative of what it takes to produce top-flight performances.

In sport, the laws of mechanics don't apply to the athlete alone. Mechanical principles are used to improve the efficiency of sport equipment and playing surfaces. Track shoes, skates, skis, and safety equipment are all designed with an understanding of the external forces that exist on earth and the muscular forces that an athlete produces. This knowledge has been instrumental in raising the standard of performance in every sport.

Technique

When we compare the performances of two athletes, we often say that one of them has better "form" or, more precisely, that one athlete has better technique. By technique we mean the pattern and sequence of movements that the athletes use to perform a sport skill, like a forearm pass in volleyball, a hip throw in judo, or a handspring in gymnastics.

Sport skills vary in number and type from one sport to the next. In some sports (e.g., discus and javelin) there is only one skill to perform. A discus thrower spins and throws the discus—nothing more. But in tennis, players have to perform forehands, backhands, volleys, and serves. Each skill, whether it's a tennis serve or a discus throw, has a specific objective determined by the rules of the sport. The tennis player wants to hit the ball over the net and into the service area in such a way that the opponent cannot return it. A discus thrower aims to throw the discus as far as possible, making sure that it lands in the designated area. Both athletes try to use good technique so that the objectives of each skill are achieved with the highest degree of efficiency and success.

Good Technique

An athlete can perform a skill with good or poor technique. Poor technique is ineffective and fails to produce the best results. You can see plenty of poor technique at any public driving range—and, along with poor technique, inferior results! Hooks and slices are mixed in with wild swings that miss the ball entirely. Even if you know little about golf, you'll be amazed by the variation you see in the performances of a single stroke. Now compare these recreational golfers with world-class players like Greg Norman, Pat Bradley, Nancy Lopez, and Fred Couples. Although Greg, Pat,

Nancy, and Fred differ in height, strength, and weight, the basic technique that they use in their strokes is the same for all four golfers. From backswing to follow-through, you'll see a smooth application of force that appears graceful and fluid. This efficiency of motion tells you that these great golfers are using good technique. Their actions are highly effective and get the job done!

The similarity in technique demonstrated by top-class golfers can also be seen when superstars like Carl Lewis, Mike Powell, and Jackie Joyner-Kersee perform the long jump. Like the elite golfers, Carl, Mike, and Jackie differ in build, speed, strength, and coordination, but they don't differ substantially in the technique they use when they perform their run-up, takeoff, flight, and landing. You'll arrive at the same conclusion when you watch great gymnasts like world-champion Shannon Miller from the United States and Vitaly Shcherbo, world all-around champion from Belarus. Although Vitaly is more muscular and powerful than Shannon, the technique they use to perform a similar skill, like a handspring or a front somersault, varies little from one gymnast to the other.

Apart from minor differences, all world-class athletes, no matter what their sport, use superior technique based on the best use of the mechanical principles that control human movement. But it's important to remember that the refined, polished movements that you see in the technique of an elite athlete seldom occur by chance. Likewise, it's virtually impossible for an athlete to reach world-class status without the assistance of someone who knows why it's better to perform the actions in a sport skill in one way rather than another. Today's top athletes get help from

Can You Recognize Superior Technique?

What are the visible characteristics of superior technique as performed by world-class athletes? Answer: an appearance of smoothness, coordination, and grace and an efficient use of all their physical abilities. Think of the fluid sprinting of Carl Lewis and Florence Griffith Joyner or the height and flight of dancer Mikhail Baryshnikov and basketball great Michael Jordan. Consider the rows of 10s awarded for the flawless performances of Greg Louganis and Nadia Comaneci or the grace of Muhammad Ali when he "floated like a butterfy and stung like a bee." The technique that these athletes used was so efficient that their performances looked effortless!

knowledgeable coaches who critically observe their performances and tell them what is efficient movement and what is not. The coach's knowledge, coupled with the athletes' talent and discipline, helps to produce a first-rate performance.

Teaching Good Technique

What must you know in order to teach good technique? As an example, let's look at what's necessary when you teach novices to drive a golf ball. When you introduce this skill, it's great if you can tee up the ball and demonstrate superb technique. It also helps if you can explain what each phase of the drive should feel like. But "show and tell" is not enough! It's important for you to know why the actions of driving a golf ball are best performed one way and not another, and to understand what is gained from stance, weight shift, hip rotation, and the extension of the arms when the ball is struck. Successful coaches pass this information on to the athletes by using progressions and coaching advice appropriate to the athlete's age and maturity.

If you coach a volleyball team or instruct classes in volleyball, like the golf coach you need to have a background in mechanics. In volleyball it's essential to know the mechanical reasons why certain movements get a player up in the air for a spike and why other movements do not! In baseball a pitching coach aims to teach the most efficient actions for the windup, delivery, and follow-through. Similarly, a batting coach works to make the batter a more effective hitter. The baseball and volleyball coaches are using their knowledge of mechanical principles when they eliminate poor movements and replace them with actions that are more efficient.

The Failure of Traditional Training Methods

There are many coaches and athletes who still follow old, traditional methods in their workouts—methods that demonstrate a lack of understanding of mechanical principles. Some people are happy using a trial-and-error method. Occasionally they get good results, but more often they don't! Many coaches will teach their athletes a technique based on a world champion's, with-

out taking into account differences in physique, training, and maturity. Similarly, young athletes will copy every action of a world-class performer, including idiosyncrasies that are mechanically ineffectual. Al Oerter, four-time Olympic champion from 1956 to 1968, frequently inverted the discus as he swung his arm back during his windup. This action was simply a personal trait, which added nothing to the mechanical efficiency of Oerter's throwing technique, yet many young athletes copied it, believing that it would add distance to their throws. Coaches and athletes who blindly mimic the methods and techniques of others progress only so far. It's much better if they can distinguish between mechanically correct movements and those that serve no purpose. *Mechanics of Sport* will help you eliminate this haphazard approach. By developing a background in mechanics you'll be able to analyze performances and teach movement patterns that produce efficient technique. This will lead to better performances.

Getting the Most From *Mechanics of Sport*

Most people involved in coaching are reluctant to study sport mechanics because from past experience they know it has meant tackling texts loaded with formulas, calculations, and scientific terminology. These texts are frequently written by academics who fail to explain the relationship of good technique to the principles of mechanics in a manner that is meaningful to coaches and sport enthusiasts. You'll be happy to find that *Mechanics of Sport* is a very different type of book! It contains no formulas or calculations, and it uses familiar measurements, like pounds, feet, and inches, while giving you metric equivalents as necessary. It doesn't matter whether you coach, teach, perform as an athlete, or merely observe this is a book that you can learn from immediately.

How *Mechanics of Sport* Will Help You

All you need in order to get the most from *Mechanics of Sport* is a desire to know how and why things work in the world of sport. In other words, if you have curiosity and a desire to improve, you'll get a lot of useful information from this text. Here's how:

• **You will learn to observe, analyze, and correct errors in performance.** This is the most important benefit that you'll get from reading *Mechanics of Sport*. This text will help you distinguish between efficient and inefficient movements in an athlete's technique. It will teach you how to pick out unproductive movements and follow up with precise instructions that help optimize performance. You won't waste time with vague advice like "Throw harder" or "Try to be more dynamic." Obscure tips like these only confuse and frustrate the athletes you're trying to help. On the other hand, if you're the athlete and your coach is not present, a basic knowledge of sport mechanics will help you understand why you should try to eliminate certain movements in your technique and emphasize other actions.

• **You'll be better able to assess the effectiveness of innovations in sport equipment.** When Greg Lemond of the United States won the Tour de France by a few seconds over Laurent Fignon of France, he proved the value of fitness and determination. But equally important, he demonstrated that the aerodynamic helmet and aerobars that he used during the final time trial were instrumental in giving him an edge over his opponent. Laurent Fignon sat up straighter on his bike and cycled bareheaded, his long hair dragging in the wind. Both Fignon and his coach should have been more aware of the advantages gained from superior aerodynamics. *Mechanics of Sport* will help you understand the wide application of aerodynamic principles not only to cycling but also to other sports like discus and javelin throwing, ski jumping, and baseball pitching. It will also give you a knowledge base that will help you assess changes and innovations that occur continuously in the world of sport. You'll be in a better position to modify your athlete's technique to take advantage of these changes. If you don't keep up, your athlete will be at a disadvantage before the competition begins.

• **You'll be better prepared to assess training methods for potential safety problems.** Think of an athlete squatting with a barbell on the shoulders. Where should your athlete position the bar? Should it be placed high on the shoulders or lower down? And what about the

angle of the athlete's back during the squatting action? What are the mechanical implications of a full squat compared with half and three-quarter squats, and how fast should the athlete lower into the squat position? If you know about levers and torque, you'll understand why it's dangerous to bend forward when you squat. Likewise, if you are familiar with the characteristics of momentum and understand how every action has an equal and opposite reaction, you'll know that dropping at high speed into a full squat puts tremendous stress on the lower back and the knees. It's possible that you have been teaching good technique but don't fully understand why one action is potentially dangerous and another is not. *Mechanics of Sport* will give you the reasons.

In gymnastics you will frequently see spotting techniques that provide a high level of safety and other techniques that endanger both the gymnast and the spotter! By reading *Mechanics of Sport* you'll understand why efficient spotting requires an understanding of balance, levers, torque, and the momentum generated by the gymnast performing the skill. The information you find in *Mechanics of Sport* will help you teach safe spotting techniques in gymnastics and good technique in weight training. Of course, *Mechanics of Sport* is not limited to these two sports. You'll find that you can apply the mechanical principles that you read about in *Mechanics of Sport* to every sport.

• **You will be better able to assess the value of innovations in the ways in which sport skills are performed.** In sport, our capacity for reasoning and creativity has been responsible for the advances that have occurred in talent selection, technique, training, and equipment design. We are all gifted with a tremendous capacity for creativity, and to be a good coach you must use this creativity to search for better ways to improve your athlete's performance. All athletes differ in physique, temperament, and physical ability, and what works for one athlete will not necessarily work for another. To help your athletes achieve top-flight performances, it's good to learn why sport techniques are performed as they are and to be prepared to modify certain aspects of these techniques when they don't fit the age, maturity, and experience of your athletes.

There are many examples of the willingness of coaches and athletes to try out new ideas. In team games, think of how coaches modify attack and defense formations relative to the team they

Never Discount Individual Creativity and Inventiveness

Just as Dick Fosbury revolutionized high jumping, so Graeme Obree from Scotland set the cycling world talking with his self-designed bike. Obree removed the crossbar, shortened the length of the bike, and reduced the width of the bottom bracket. With no crossbar and with the pedals closer together, he cycled with his legs brushing against each other. His chest lay flat and horizontal on top of the handlebars. Obree's strange bike and awkward-looking technique reduced air resistance to a minimum. Although lying with the chest on the handlebars was subsequently outlawed, Obree was not to be beaten by changes in the rules. He modified his bike even further to cycle without his chest contacting the handlebars but with his upper body stretched forward like an arrow. Training, determination, and an understanding of mechanics helped make Obree world champion in 1993.

will face in an upcoming contest. Among athletes, think of how the creativity and experimentation of Dick Fosbury revolutionized the high jump, and how the glide-and-rotary technique has increased the distances thrown in the shot put. In gymnastics, consider how many skills have been named after their inventors (like the "Thomas Flair," named after America's great gymnast, Kurt Thomas). So don't stagnate: Be curious and learn the how and why of technique. At the same time, be creative and willing to experiment—and be sure to encourage your athletes to use their own creative capacities as well. Always look for ways to improve your understanding of the sport you are coaching. Be an analyst and innovator at the same time!

• **You will know what to expect from different body types and different levels of maturity.** If you understand the mechanical principles governing the technique of your sport, you'll understand why young athletes who are growing fast have a tough time maneuvering, changing direction, and coordinating their movements. You'll realize that you cannot and should not expect young athletes to follow the same training regimens that are comfortable for mature athletes. You'll also understand why tall athletes with long arms and legs have an edge in some sports but are at a disadvantage in others. Similarly, you will realize why smaller athletes tend to have a good strength-to-weight ratio and can cut, turn, and shift more quickly than athletes who are taller and heavier.

How *Mechanics of Sport* Is Organized

Mechanics of Sport is divided into two parts, each with a different focus.

Part I contains chapters 1 through 6. Chapter 1 is an overview of what you'll find in *Mechanics of Sport*. It's titled "Making a Smart Move" because it *is* a smart move for you to develop a background in sport mechanics.

The next five chapters get into the meat of sport mechanics. They have purposely been given some informal titles, like "Starting With Basics," "Getting a Move On," "Rocking and Rolling," "Don't Be a Pushover," and "Going With the Flow." You'll understand why these titles were chosen when you read about the various forces at work as athletes perform in their sports. These chapters explain the interaction between an athlete, the athlete's equipment, and the ever-present external forces that assist or oppose the athlete during the performance of a sport skill. You'll learn what forces are at work when sprinters accelerate, gymnasts spin in the air, and pitchers hurl curveballs. You'll understand the mechanics of good swimming technique and what advantages and disadvantages exist when athletes compete at high altitudes.

In part II, chapters 7 and 8 explain how you can put to work the information you learned in part I. These chapters discuss why athletes must make their muscles work as a team and why it's so important to synchronize and coordinate muscle actions. It is this synchronization and coordination of muscle action that produces superior technique—technique that has resulted in a 20 ft pole vault, an 8 ft high jump, and a long jump close to 30 ft.

Chapters 7 and 8 are particularly useful to coaches and to physical educators because they explain how to observe and analyze an athlete's technique and how to set about correcting errors that are found. Each chapter gives you a series of steps to follow. You'll learn how to break a skill down into phases and what to look for as you analyze each phase. Then you'll read a series of important mechanical principles, which you can refer to when you start correcting errors.

In chapter 9 you'll study the technique and mechanics in a wide range of sport skills that include sprinting, jumping, swimming, lifting, throwing, and kicking. First you'll read descriptions of the most prominent features in the performance of these skills. Then you'll read the mechanical reasons why the technique of the skill is best performed in a certain way. The goal in this chapter is to show you how technique and mechanics are inseparable, no matter what the sport.

Mechanics of Sport finishes with a glossary and a list of references that help you expand your knowledge of sport mechanics. The glossary avoids dull scientific explanations. Instead it relates scientific principles to athletes and to the movement of sport implements, like bats, balls, and javelins.

After you've read *Mechanics of Sport*, you'll be able to watch an athletic performance and know immediately what external forces the athlete has to contend with. You'll be able to analyze an athlete's movements and immediately recognize how they can be improved. You'll spot poor actions and replace them with efficient movements that form quality technique—technique based on sound mechanical principles.

Understanding how physical laws influence sport performances will help you, whether you are coaching, competing, or simply watching as a spectator. If you coach remember that sport mechanics is just one tool that you'll use. You'll also need to improve your knowledge in such areas as sport psychology, physiology, nutrition, sport injuries, and the teaching of sport skills. The American Sport Education Program can provide you with all the necessary information in these areas.

REVIEW QUESTIONS

1. What kind of research are scientists interested in who work in the field of mechanics?

2. Explain a common weakness with traditional methods of coaching.

3. How will you benefit from having an understanding of sport mechanics when you correct errors in skill performance?

4. As you watch a sport skill being performed, you notice that elite athletes perform the *basic technique* of this skill in a similar manner. What is the reason for elite athletes performing the basic technique of the skill in a similar manner?

5. Occasionally new methods of performing a skill are developed by creative athletes and coaches. How will a knowledge of sport mechanics help you to assess the efficiency of these methods?

6. What are the visible characteristics of efficient technique as performed by a world-class athlete?

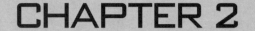 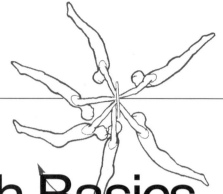

CHAPTER 2

Starting With Basics

When you finish reading this chapter, you should be able to explain

- how gravity affects athletic performance;

- the relationship between body weight, mass, and inertia;

- how the center of gravity of an athlete or an object can vary in position;

- the difference between speed, velocity, and acceleration;

- how athletes make use of the earth's reaction force;

- how athletes make use of force vectors;

- the difference between linear, angular, and general motion; and

- the factors that influence the flight paths of athletes or objects (such as baseballs and javelins).

In this chapter we'll look at some basic mechanical concepts. We will discuss the effect of the earth's gravitational pull. Even though the force of gravity can help an athlete, in many sports (e.g., jumping and throwing), **gravity** is also the toughest opposition that the athlete has to face. So it's worthwhile knowing as much as you can about the characteristics of this ever-present force. You'll learn in this chapter how an athlete's body mass and body weight are related and what is meant by inertia. You'll see that a massive athlete has more inertia than one who has less body mass. Like gravity, inertia can be helpful in some sport skills, but in others it presents real problems for an athlete. You'll understand how every action has an equal and opposite reaction, and you'll read some examples of how this law influences sport skills.

Chapter 2 concludes with a discussion of the factors that affect the trajectories followed by athletes, and objects like balls, discuses, and javelins. The discussion of trajectories brings you back again to the ever-present force of gravity and the part it plays in determining the shape of the flight path that athletes and objects follow. Be sure to note how all the mechanical concepts discussed in this chapter interrelate, and watch for this interrelationship to continue in later chapters.

Body Weight

Athletes who want to perform well in their chosen events monitor their body weight. They know that too much or too little weight can affect performance. For all of us, checking our body weight is a means of assessing our general health and fitness.

When we get on a scale the dial gives us a reading that we associate with the amount of body mass (i.e., bones, muscle, fat, tissue) that we carry around. A common assumption is that an athlete's body weight squashes the springs in the scale, the readout on the dial representing the amount that the springs are compressed. This is true, but what actually happens is a little more complex.

In mechanical terms an athlete's **weight** represents the earth's gravitational force pulling on the athlete's body, and vice versa, the pull of the athlete's body on the earth! The readout on the scale represents how much pull exists between the two. The earth pulls the athlete downward and, in reverse, the athlete pulls the earth upward.

The degree of attraction, or pull, between the athlete and the earth depends on how much mass the earth has, and how much body mass the athlete has. The more attraction, the more the springs of the scale are compressed. So an athlete with more body mass compresses the springs to a greater extent than an athlete who has less body mass. As a result the needle on the scale moves farther around the dial.

Mass

What do we mean by body mass, or, more specifically, the word mass? **Mass** simply means "substance" or "matter." If an object has substance and occupies space it has mass. What's more important, if it has mass it can attract and pull on other objects that have mass too. Athletes are made up of muscles, bones, fat, tissues, and fluids, all of which are substance or **matter** and have mass. So an athlete, having mass, pulls on the earth, and the earth, having mass as well, pulls on the athlete.

A wrestler in the heavyweight division has more mass than a lightweight gymnast. The attraction between the earth and the heavyweight wrestler is greater than between the earth and the gymnast. It shows up on the scale. The needle on the scale may point to 220 lb for the wrestler and 80 lb for the gymnast. In metric measurements, the wrestler will weigh 100 kg and the gymnast 36.2 kg.

How Weight and Mass Are Related

The earth's gravitational pull radiates from its core much like the ripples of a stone thrown in a pond. The closer you are to the earth's core, the stronger its pull. Because the earth is not perfectly round, an athlete is farther from the core standing at the equator than standing at the North or South Pole. As a result an athlete, or an implement like a javelin, will weigh a little less at the equator than at either Pole. If the athlete climbed to the top of a mountain at the equator, she would be farther from the earth's core, and her weight would be reduced even more. We must also consider two additional items: the earth's daily rotation around its axis and the fact that the earth's spin causes it to bulge outward at the equator and flatten out at the Poles. This means that the closer you are to the equator, the larger the rotary pathway you travel around as the earth turns on its axis. As a result, an athlete or an object at the equator travels more than 1,000 miles an hour faster than at the North or South Pole! The faster you travel during the earth's daily rotation, the more your body mass tries to fly out and away from the earth's surface. You don't take off into space of course, but the body's increased outward pull fights against gravity's inward attraction. This characteristic also causes you to weigh a little less than you would at the Poles.

Consider the result of all these factors: An athlete who weighs 200 lb at the Poles will weigh about 198.94 lb at sea level at the equator, and an athlete who weighs 200 lb at sea level will weigh approximately 199.77 lb at an altitude of 12,000 ft. These small changes in poundage tell us that an athlete's body weight is a function of variations in the earth's gravitational pull on the athlete's mass. An athlete's body *mass* can remain constant, yet the same person's body *weight* can fluctuate, depending on where the athlete is on the earth. The same principle applies to the weight of a shot, a javelin, or any kind of equipment used in a sporting contest.

Be sure to understand the relationship between weight and mass. Although weight and mass are different, this difference is not too important in sport, because most sport skills take place on or close to the surface of the earth. Under these conditions weight and mass experience the same proportions (i.e., an athlete who weighs more than another athlete will also have more mass).

Inertia

The word **inertia** means resistance to action or to change. We use the word inertia in everyday life to characterize people who are slow to commit themselves to action. So in everyday life there's a relationship between inertia and laziness.

In mechanical terms, inertia means more than just laziness because it describes the desire of an object to continue doing whatever it's doing—even when it's moving. All objects (and it doesn't matter whether they are athletes or equipment like clubs, bats, or balls) want to remain motionless. But if a force is great enough to make them move in a particular direction, they want to continue moving in the same direction at a constant speed.

How Mass Is Related to Inertia

Once on the move, the more mass an object has, the greater its desire to keep moving. Other forces get into the act, of course, so that on earth a constant speed seldom occurs for any length of time.

Air resistance, the pull of gravity, friction, and the forces applied by opponents are examples of the opposition that slows and finally halts an athlete or an object that's on the move.

The more massive and heavy an athlete, the more the athlete's body mass resists change. So a giant 300 lb athlete has to produce great muscular force to get his body mass moving. Once moving in a particular direction, the athlete must produce an immense amount of muscular force to stop or to change direction. This means that athletes with less body mass have less inertia and need to apply less force to get themselves going. Likewise, they need less force than a more massive athlete to maneuver or stop themselves, once they're on the move.

One of the best examples of inertia at work occurs in football. Quarterbacks are protected by offensive linemen, who are immense and have tremendous mass. It takes an incredible amount of force to move these linemen out of the way. But offensive linemen face equally enormous defensive linemen whose job it is to get through their protective wall and harass the quarterback. In this scenario the offensive linemen represent inertia at rest and the defensive linemen represent inertia on the move.

The massive size of offensive and defensive linemen is one example of inertia being used to advantage. But if you take these giant football players and put them in a sport like squash or badminton, their mass and inertia work against them. It's no good having tremendous mass when sudden and varied movement changes are required *unless* you have the strength to move your mass quickly and to control it once it's moving. Most massive athletes have a poorer strength to weight ratio than smaller, less massive athletes, so they have a harder time stopping, starting, and changing direction. That's why badminton and squash players are lean, lightweight, and anything but massive! If you're a small, lightweight squash player, you can get a lot of pleasure from making your massive opponent crash into the side walls! You have a friend helping you in the court—your opponent's inertia!

An interesting example of inertia at work occurs when athletes are in flight. Consider two thrill seekers who decide to bungee jump from a bridge. One is twice as massive as the other. They step off the bridge at the same instant. Surprisingly, both accelerate toward the earth at approximately the same rate. Because the earth attracts the more massive bungee jumper twice as much, you might think that he will accelerate downward twice as fast. But he has twice the inertia and so resists being accelerated by gravity twice as much! In this situation air resistance plays a negligible role and both thrill seekers accelerate downward at approximately the same rate.

Think of inertia as an enemy when an athlete wants to get moving, because the inertia of the athlete's body mass resists acceleration. Once on the move, inertia can be an athlete's friend because inertia wants to keep the athlete going! The difference between "resting" and "moving" inertia causes athletes to expend much more energy at the start of a 100m dash than when sprinting in the middle of the race. The two characteristics of inertia, to resist and then persist, do not only occur in linear situations where objects and athletes move in a straight line. They also occur in rotary situations where objects like bats and clubs are swung, and where athletes like divers and gymnasts somersault and twist.

Speed, Acceleration, and Velocity

In describing the two bungee jumpers, we talked of their acceleration as they fell toward the earth. Let's make sure that we understand the difference between speed and acceleration, and then introduce *velocity*—a term that you'll find frequently throughout this text.

If an elite sprinter runs 100 m in 10 sec, we know that the athlete has run a certain distance (100 m) in a particular time (10 sec). From this information you can work out the sprinter's average speed, which is 35 km/h or 22.36 mph (22.36 mph = 10.9 yd/sec).

22.36 mph is the **speed** that the sprinter *averaged* over a distance of 100 m—nothing else. These numbers don't tell you the sprinter's top speed, nor do they tell you anything about the sprinter's **acceleration**. A sprinter who averages 22.36 mph over 100 m runs faster and slower than 22.36 mph during different phases of the race. Why? Because immediately after the start the athlete is gaining speed and for a while runs much slower than 22.36 mph. The athlete then has to run faster somewhere else in the race to average 22.36 mph over the whole distance.

If you had a radar gun like those that baseball scouts use to find the speed of a pitcher's fastball, it could feed back to you the rate at which the athlete accelerates after coming out of the blocks. The gun will help determine over what distance the athlete holds a particular speed, and it will help you assess by how much the athlete slows, or decelerates, at the end of the race.

Rates of acceleration vary dramatically from one athlete to another. Some athletes rocket out of the blocks and have tremendous acceleration over the first 40 m. Thereafter their acceleration rate drops off, and close to the tape they may even decelerate. Athletes who raced against Olympic champion Carl Lewis were well aware that he could still be accelerating at the 70 m mark in the 100m dash. His rate of acceleration may have been less than his opponents at the start, but his acceleration continued longer. Over the last 30 m Carl frequently caught and passed athletes who were tying up and struggling to hold their form!

It is important to realize that an athlete can reduce the rate of acceleration and still increase speed. As long as acceleration exists, even if it's minimal, speed will increase. If deceleration occurs, speed will be reduced. How much an athlete's speed increases or reduces depends on the rate of acceleration and deceleration.

Uniform acceleration and **uniform deceleration** mean that an athlete or an object speeds up or slows at a regular rate. An example of uniform acceleration occurs when a four-man toboggan slides down a slope and accelerates to a speed of 15 ft/sec by the first second, 30 ft/sec by the second second, and 45 ft/sec by the third second. For every second that the toboggan is moving it is increasing speed at a uniform rate of 15 ft/sec. You write this acceleration as 15 ft/sec/sec or 15 ft/sec^2. Notice that there is one distance unit (i.e., 15 ft) and two time units (i.e., sec/sec) whenever you refer to acceleration. This indicates the rate of change of speed, or the amount of speed added (i.e., 15 ft/sec) with each successive time unit (i.e., 1 sec) that passes. If the toboggan decelerates at a uniform rate, then the reverse occurs. It is slowing or losing speed at a uniform rate.

Uniform acceleration and deceleration don't happen that often in sport. When athletes (and objects like balls or javelins) are on the move, varying forces such as friction and air resistance affect them, and these forces cause their acceleration (or deceleration) to be varied (or nonuniform). However, one of the best examples that we have of uniform acceleration and deceleration occurs in flights of short duration such as those in diving and gymnastics. In these situations air resistance is negligible. Gravity uniformly slows or decelerates the athletes as they rise in flight by a speed of 32 ft/sec for every sec of flight (i.e., 32 ft/sec^2) and accelerates them at a uniform rate of 32 ft/sec^2 on the way down. (In the metric system 32 ft/sec^2 = 9.8 m/sec^2.) Sometimes you'll see deceleration described as **negative acceleration** and acceleration called **positive acceleration**. A minus sign in front of 32 ft/sec^2 (i.e., -32 ft/sec^2) indicates that the diver is decelerating at a rate of 32 ft/sec for each second that the diver is rising in the air.

How does the word **velocity** fit into this description of speed, acceleration, and deceleration? Velocity is nothing more than a more precise description of speed. It means both speed and direction. For example, 20 mph simply indicates speed; 20 mph due south indicates velocity. Speed tells you how fast. Velocity tells you how fast and in what direction.

How Gravity Affects Athletic Performance

Earlier in this chapter, we saw how the earth's gravitational pull varies. How do these differences in the earth's gravitational pull affect athletic performance? Athletes experienced slightly less gravitational pull at the 1968 Olympics in Mexico City, which is at higher altitude and closer to the equator, than at the 1952 Olympics in Helsinki or the 1980 Games in Moscow, both of which are in northern latitudes and close to sea level. Considering gravity by itself, and not air resistance, Peter Brancazio, an avid sports fan and physics professor at Brooklyn College, calculated that a 70 ft shot put in Oslo, Norway (latitude 60 degrees N), would travel 70 ft 1 inch in Montreal, Canada (45 degrees N), 70 ft 2 inch in Cairo, Egypt (30 degrees N), and 70 ft 3 inch in Caracas, Venezuela (10 degrees N). A 300 ft javelin throw in Moscow (56 degrees N) would travel 301 ft in Lima, Peru (12 degrees S).

Of greater importance than the slight reduction in gravity's pull is the thin air that occurs at high altitude. It had great effect on the athletes who competed at Mexico City. In thin air less oxygen is available than at sea level. This means that athletes have to breathe more often to get the oxygen they need. This can seriously affect distance runners but does not affect athletes in short sprints who run on stored energy supplies in their bodies. When Bob Beamon set his world record in the long jump in Mexico City, he benefited from a slight reduction in gravity, reduced air resistance from the thin air (as he sprinted down the runway), and the fact that his approach was a short sprint and not a distance run.

After standing for many years, Beamon's record was beaten by Mike Powell in the 1991 World Track and Field Championships in Tokyo. Tokyo is at a much lower altitude than Mexico City. One can assume that Powell's jump in Tokyo would have produced a greater distance had he performed it in Mexico City. Additional proof of the assistance of altitude occurred at a track meet at high altitude in Italy in 1995 when Cuban Ivan Pedrosa jumped a single centimeter (4/10 of an inch) farther than Mike Powell's four-year-old record.

The Effect of Zero Gravity

What happens to our bodies when there is no gravity? In space an astronaut's bones suffer mineral loss and become weaker. Blood pools in the upper body, and this causes a shift in the astronaut's center of gravity. The astronaut's balance is also disturbed. The cardiovascular system weakens and muscles accustomed to fighting gravity lose strength. When Russian cosmonauts returned to earth after a year in space, they had to be helped out of the capsule because they couldn't stand. The cosmonauts even found the weight of blankets uncomfortable. It took a long time to become reaccustomed to the earth's gravitational force.

The Acceleration of Gravity

When a pole-vaulter drops from above the bar, gravity accelerates the athlete toward the pit. If the athlete clears the bar at 20 ft rather than 15 ft, the extra distance gives the earth more time to accelerate the athlete downward. Dropping from 20 ft, a pole-vaulter hits the pit at a greater velocity than when clearing 15 ft.

The pole-vaulter's acceleration toward the earth is similarly experienced by a tower diver heading toward the water. Because of earth's gravitational pull, a diver continuously accelerates during the fall to the water. Figure 2.1 shows an athlete diving from a very high tower that is 256 ft up. After 1 sec of fall, the athlete is traveling at a velocity of 32 ft per sec or 21.8 mph. After 2 sec, the athlete's velocity has reached 64 ft per sec or 43.6 mph. At the 3 sec mark, the athlete has reached 96 ft per sec or 65.4 mph. Finally at the 4 sec mark, the athlete's velocity has increased to an incredible 128 ft per sec or 87.2 mph! Because of the regular addition of 32 ft per sec or 21.8 mph for every second, we say that the force of gravity uniformly accelerates a falling athlete by a velocity of 32 ft/sec for every second of fall, or 32 ft/sec^2.

How can you get some idea of the incredible acceleration of gravity? Look again at Figure 2.1 and check the distance the athlete covers with each second of fall. After 1 sec the athlete has fallen 16 ft. This is not very far, but gravity has only had 1 sec to accelerate the athlete from zero. By the 2 sec mark, the athlete has fallen a distance of 64 ft. At the 3 sec mark the athlete has reached 144 ft, and finally by 4 sec the distance covered is a colossal 256 ft. The athlete accelerates downward at a uniform rate of 32 ft/sec^2 and so with each passing second, the athlete is adding on an additional 21.8 mph. Because of the tremendous increase in velocity, the athlete covers increasingly large stretches of distance with each second that passes.

The phenomenal acceleration caused by gravity's pull tells you why tower diving is a risky sport. The tower is 10 m (i.e., just under 33 ft) from the surface of the water. Tower divers take about 1.75 sec to reach the surface of the water and are traveling at close to 38 mph when they enter! Water is hard when you hit it traveling at that velocity!

Does the uniform acceleration of springboard and tower divers mean that a parachutist in a free

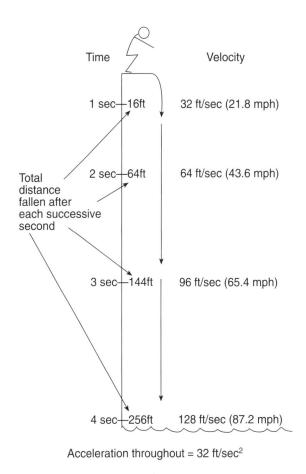

Time / Velocity

1 sec — 16ft   32 ft/sec (21.8 mph)

Total distance fallen after each successive second

2 sec — 64ft   64 ft/sec (43.6 mph)

3 sec — 144ft   96 ft/sec (65.4 mph)

4 sec — 256ft   128 ft/sec (87.2 mph)

Acceleration throughout = 32 ft/sec^2

Fig. 2.1.   Distance, velocity, and acceleration due to gravity. (Air resistance has been discounted.)

fall from several thousand feet up accelerates continuously toward the earth? No, because in a free fall a parachutist falls for a much longer time than a diver. Air resistance in the denser atmosphere close to the earth's surface increases to a point at which the parachutist falls at a constant (or terminal) velocity of about 150 mph. Free fall velocities in excess of 600 mph have been recorded at extreme altitudes where the atmosphere is really thin and where the air resistance to acceleration is minimal.

An Athlete's Center of Gravity

The earth's gravitational pull is one of the biggest oppositional forces that the athlete fights. To get up in the air as high as possible, to maintain one's stability and equilibrium, to throw far, all require an understanding of how this ever-present force operates.

Cliff Divers Respect Gravity's Acceleration

Cliff divers in Acapulco, Mexico dive from 118 ft and hit the water at close to 60 mph—more than double the top speed reached by an Olympic sprinter in the 100 m dash! The extra distance that the divers fall gives gravity more time to accelerate them. Moreover, to clear the cliff face on the way down, divers must thrust outward in excess of 20 ft. They time their entries into the water so that incoming waves make the water deep enough. Failure can mean hitting the coral a mere 16 ft below the surface!

The earth's gravitational pull on an athlete is concentrated at the athlete's **center of gravity**. The same applies for any object that comes within range of the earth's gravitational pull. It doesn't matter whether the athlete is standing still or moving from one body position to another, the earth's gravitational pull is always concentrated at the athlete's center of gravity.

Before we look at an athlete's center of gravity, let's consider a shot that is perfectly spherical and made up of the same substance (iron) throughout. The earth pulls equally on every iron particle that makes up the shot. If you could add all these "pulls" and combine them into a single resultant force, the place where this force would act is the shot's center of gravity. In a perfectly spherical iron shot, the center of gravity is dead center in the shot (i.e., equidistant in any direction from its surface). You'd find as much mass directly above the shot's center as directly below, and likewise to the left compared to the right.

Here's another example. Imagine a 12 in ruler that is 1 in across. You could balance this ruler like a seesaw on your fingertip at a point 6 inches in from the ends and 1/2 inches in from the sides. This spot would be directly below the ruler's center of gravity. There would be equal amounts of the ruler's mass lengthwise and widthwise from the ruler's center of gravity. This is why it balances on your fingertip.

An athlete's body differs from a shot and from a 12 in ruler because it is not made of the same material throughout nor is the athlete's body mass uniformly distributed from head to foot. Instead the athlete's body is made up of different shapes and substances like bone, muscle, fat, and tissue, all of which differ in density. Bone and muscle are more dense than fat and so have more mass "squashed" into the space they occupy. The earth attracts and pulls more on those parts of the athlete's body that have more mass than the parts that have less mass. This means that the athlete's center of gravity is not necessarily central and equidistant in all directions from the surface of the athlete like the iron shot that we described. If an athlete has more mass in the torso and upper body than in the legs, then the athlete's center of gravity will be positioned more toward the upper body. If the athlete has more mass in the legs, the reverse occurs. Even though the athlete's center of gravity is not equidistant from all surfaces of the athlete, the athlete's body mass is balanced around her center of gravity. Just like the shot there will be as much mass directly above the athlete's center of gravity as there is directly below, and as much mass to the left of the athlete's center of gravity as there is to the right.

Locating an Athlete's Center of Gravity

Where is an athlete's center of gravity? For most adult male athletes standing with the arms by the sides, the center of gravity is approximately at belt level or about an inch above the navel. For female athletes the center of gravity is slightly lower. The reason for the difference is that males tend to have more body mass in the shoulders and less in the hips, whereas for females the reverse occurs.

Shifting the Center Of Gravity

An athlete's center of gravity seldom stays in the same place for any length of time. Even when sleeping, the slightest shift in body position also redistributes the athlete's body mass. Consequently, the athlete's center of gravity moves as well.

If an athlete stands erect and then moves a leg forward to take a step, the athlete's center of gravity shifts in the same direction. If the athlete moves the leg plus an arm, the center of gravity shifts forward even farther because more mass has been moved.

The distance that an athlete's center of gravity moves depends on how much of the athlete's body mass is moved and how far it's moved. Legs are heavy and have a lot of mass, so they cause a greater shift in the center of gravity than when moving one arm by itself. Flexing at the waist shifts the center of gravity as does tilting the head. The shift of the center of gravity always relates to the amount of mass that's moved and the dis-

tance that it is moved (see Figure 2.2).

What happens if the athlete holds a bat in her hands, or hoists a heavy barbell over her head? In both situations, consider the combined center of gravity of the athlete's mass with the mass of the implement. Hoisting a heavy barbell to arm's length above the head shifts the combined center of gravity upward a long way because the large mass of the barbell has been moved vertically a large distance. In addition, the athlete has raised the mass of the arms above the head as well. The longer and more massive the athlete's arms and the more massive the barbell, the farther the combined center of gravity will move (see Figure 2.3).

If the athlete no longer holds the barbell, then the center of gravity reestablishes itself relative to the athlete's body position. So if the athlete

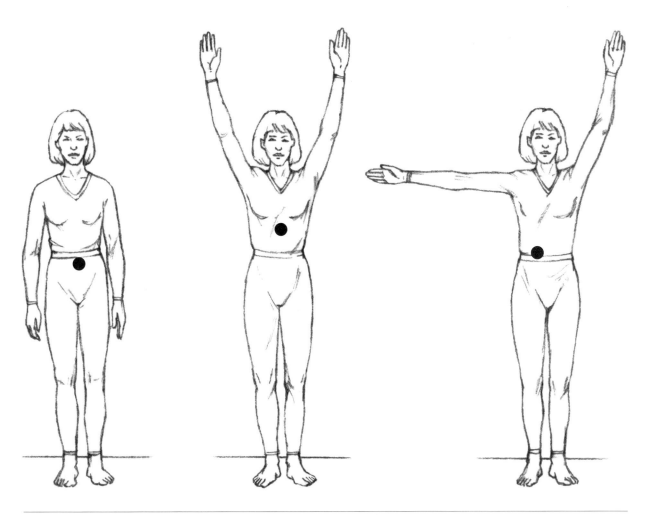

Fig. 2.2. An athlete's center of gravity shifts as the body's position changes.

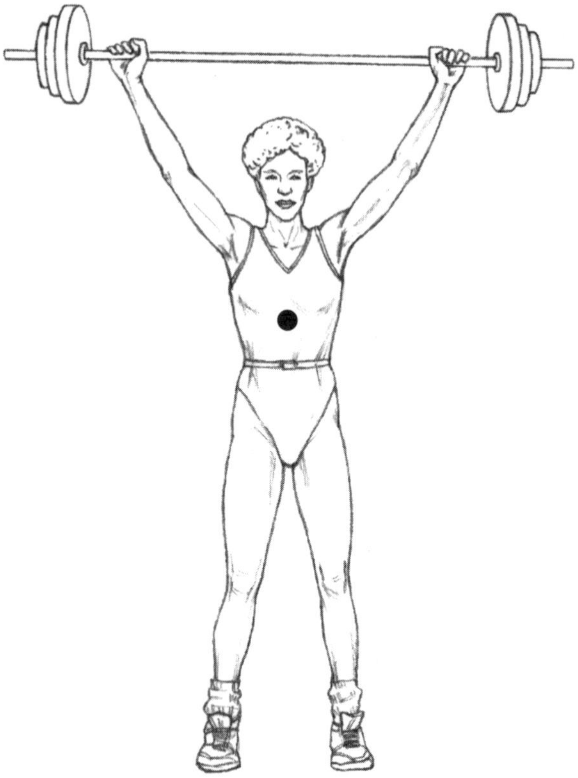

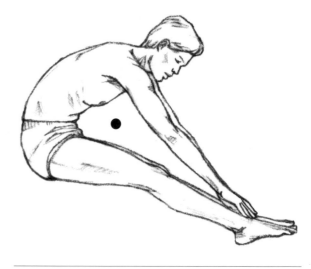

Fig. 2.4. Center of gravity for a diver in a piked position.

Fig. 2.3. Combined center of gravity of an athlete with a heavy barbell overhead.

lowers the arms, her center of gravity moves downward as well. The barbell, of course, will have a center of gravity of its own.

Is it possible to shift the center of gravity outside the body? Yes, and the more flexible the athlete the easier it is. A diver performing a toe touch in a piked position reaches forward with the arms and flexes at the waist. This causes the athlete's center of gravity to move forward to a position where it is no longer within the body (see Figure 2.4).

A gymnast performing a high back arch, or a back walkover, also shifts the center of gravity into a position where it is temporarily outside the body. The center of gravity moves in relation to the shift in the mass of the legs, the upper body, and the arms. The more extreme the arch, the greater the shift of the center of gravity (see Figure 2.5).

A gymnast's back arch position is much like the draped layout position a flop high jumper uses when clearing the bar. A highly flexible athlete can make his center of gravity pass under the bar while the athlete's body snakes its way

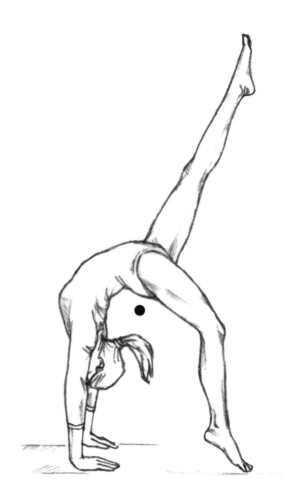

Fig. 2.5. Center of gravity during a back walkover.

over the top. The benefit of this draped bar clearance technique can be easily understood if the same athlete clears the bar using a squat jump rather than the flop technique. If the athlete clears 6 ft using the flop technique it would be necessary for the athlete to raise his center of gravity close to 8 ft to clear the same height using a squat jump (see Figure 2.6).

How Gravity Affects Flight

An athlete who is in flight has a center of gravity just as an athlete who is in contact with the earth. Body movements in the air reposition the center of gravity relative to the athlete's body movements in the same way they do on earth. On earth, an athlete tends to forget gravity's pull, until the athlete is tackled, trips, or falls! In the air the effect of the pull of gravity is really apparent. A diver propelled upward from a springboard is immediately decelerated by gravity on the way up and accelerated on the way down. As we noticed earlier, gravity decelerates the diver at the same rate on the way up as it accelerates the diver on the way down.

When an athlete is in flight, gravity concentrates its pull at the athlete's center of gravity. It makes no difference whether the athlete assumes a somersaulting position or flies through the air totally out of control with arms and legs flailing wildly! Moving the arms and legs in flight continuously repositions the center of gravity just as on the ground, but the earth still concentrates its pull at the athlete's center of gravity. Likewise, the earth concentrates its pull on the center of gravity of inanimate objects like javelins, shots, and basketballs. The big difference between these objects and athletes is that athletes can alter their shape at will while in flight. Most inanimate objects stay pretty much the same shape.

Gravity always pulls at a diver's center of gravity, but this doesn't stop them from extending their bodies and pulling themselves into a tight tuck. A tight tuck causes divers to spin faster, but

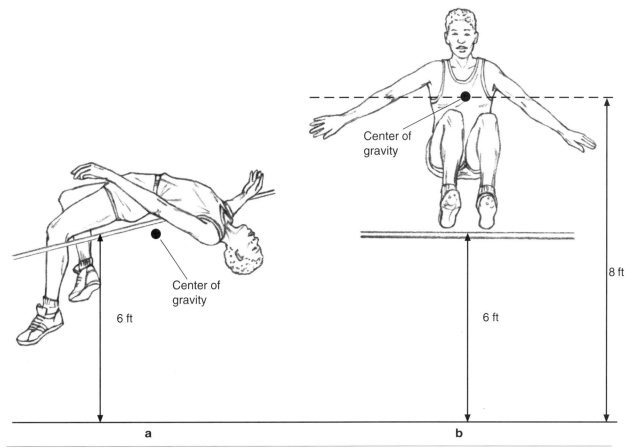

Fig. 2.6. Height that an athlete's center of gravity must be raised to clear a 6 ft bar using (a) the flop technique or (b) a squat jump.
Figure 2.6b is adapted from Dyson 1986.

this doesn't alter gravity's continued pull at their center of gravity. In chapter 4 you'll learn what causes divers and gymnasts to spin faster and what factors control their rate of spin.

In events in which the athlete is in flight for a short time (e.g., high jump, long jump, gymnastics, skating, and diving), the athlete sets the flight path of the center of gravity at takeoff. It's impossible for the athlete to alter this parabolic (i.e., curved) flight path once in the air. So if a diver makes the mistake of thrusting straight up from the board, there's nothing that can be done to avoid coming back down on the board again! Waving the arms and legs around will not change this flight path. Even great divers like Greg Louganis have been punished for a flight path that was too close to the board!

How Variations in Density Can Shift the Center of Gravity

Density refers to the amount of substance (or mass) that an athlete or an object has "squashed" into the space that they occupy. The more mass compressed into the space the more dense the athlete or the object becomes. Among metals, iron is less dense than lead, and a 16 lb shot made of iron is larger and occupies more space than a 16 lb shot made of lead. Some of the cheaper barbell sets available today have plates made of substances other than iron or steel. Usually they're coated with plastic and have a concretelike substance inside. This material is not particularly dense and so the plates tend to be huge and unwieldy. More expensive iron and steel equipment is less cumbersome because the same weight of steel or iron occupies less space.

In the human body, bone and muscle are more dense than fat. So it is possible for a small muscular athlete to have more mass and weigh more than an athlete who appears bigger but has less muscle and more fat.

Because muscle is more dense than fat, bodybuilders who spend a disproportionate time developing their upper body will increase muscle mass in this area of their body. This means that they will also raise their center of gravity. Athletes who have a high center of gravity can be at a disadvantage in sports (e.g., wrestling and judo)

where stability is at a premium. It's no different for a weight lifter with a 200 lb barbell at arm's length above the head. The mass of the 200 lb barbell raises the combined center of gravity of the weight lifter and barbell far higher than if a 100 lb barbell is raised to the same position. Athletes with a high center of gravity, including the weight lifter, have to fight harder to maintain their balance.

In chapter 5 we will discuss stability and balance and give you reasons why athletes with a high center of gravity can be at a disadvantage in maneuvering, changing direction, and defending themselves in contact sports. When we discuss buoyancy in chapter 6 you'll notice how differences in density can make one athlete a sinker and another athlete a floater.

How the Reaction Force of the Earth Acts on Athletes

Because of the attraction of their mass to other objects that have mass, athletes standing on the ground pull upward on the earth and at the same time are pulled by the earth's gravitational force toward the earth's core. The more massive the athlete, the stronger the pull. This means that an athlete presses down against the surface of the earth with a force equal to the athlete's weight. Strange as this may seem, the earth reacts to the athlete's weight by pushing upward against the athlete with an equal and opposite force. The earth pushes up with the same amount of force and in the opposite direction that the athlete's weight is pushing downward. You can think of the athlete's "weight-force" as the action and the force pushing upward as the reaction. They're equal and they oppose each other.

The force pushing up against the athlete is called a **ground reaction force**. This is an example of the familiar principle that tells us that every action has an equal and opposite reaction. If you push, press, or hit something, it's going to do the same back to you! So an unhappy player who punches a locker after a poor game actually gets punched back by the locker! Don't worry if this example is difficult to visualize. In subsequent chapters we'll return to this important principle.

When an athlete stands motionless on the earth's surface, the downward force exerted by the athlete and the upward force exerted by the earth cancel each other out. So the athlete doesn't go anywhere. The athlete can be happy about this because if there was no upward force from the earth reacting to the athlete's weight, the athlete would be constantly pulled downward toward the earth's core!

The magnitude (i.e., size) of the earth's reaction force pushing against the athlete depends on how much the athlete pushes against the ground. So the earth's reaction force depends not only on how heavy the athlete is, but also on whatever movements the athlete makes. For example, in Figure 2.7 an athlete is landing at the end of a long jump. In this situation the athlete exerts considerable force on the earth. The earth responds with an equal force on the athlete.

The forces of an athlete pushing down and the earth pushing back are crucial in determining how much friction occurs between the athlete and the earth's surface. Friction is necessary for traction, and traction is essential for movement.

In all sports, how much friction and traction are required depend on what the athlete wants to do. Sometimes an athlete wants friction and traction to be maximal and at other times the athlete wants it to be minimal. An excellent example of this variation in frictional requirement occurs in skiing. Skiers talk of "weighting and unweighting" their skis. Extending the legs and pressing downward weights the skis and pushes them down onto the snow. In reaction the force of the earth pushing up is also increased. The result is that the skis are driven into tight contact with the snow and this increases friction. Flexing the legs by pulling them upward toward the chest unweights the skis. This action lessens the force pushing downward and the earth reduces its force pushing up. As a result the friction between the ski and the snow is reduced. Weighting and unweighting the skis at the right moment helps a skier perform turns and similar maneuvers more easily. In mogul competitions, weighting and unweighting the skis occurs in rapid succession.

In flight, the reaction force from the earth no longer affects an athlete, and as a result an athlete will feel weightless. When a pole-vaulter or a diver drops downward, the earth's gravitational force accelerates every part of the athlete toward the earth at the same rate. No one part of the body feels heavier than another. The sense of the weight of the arms or the legs, which occurs when in contact with the ground, will not be apparent in flight.

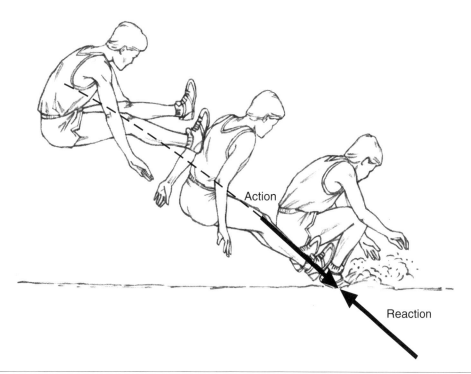

Fig. 2.7.   Action and reaction in the long jump. The action is the athlete landing; the reaction is the earth pushing back equally and in opposition to the athlete.

Without the earth to push against, an athlete in flight really notices how every action has an equal and opposite reaction. Move part of the body this way and another part moves in the opposing direction. It's impossible to stop this force-counterforce relationship even if the athlete wanted to do so. Can you see and experience this force-counterforce relationship on the ground? Yes, it's quite easy! Sit upright in a swivel chair with your feet off the ground. Extend both arms horizontally in front of your body. Then swing both arms vigorously to the left. You'll find that your legs and lower body rotate to the right. Your arm movement is the action, and the movement of your legs is the reaction. Figure 2.8 shows this action and reaction performed on a special turntable designed to have very little friction and so it moves easily.

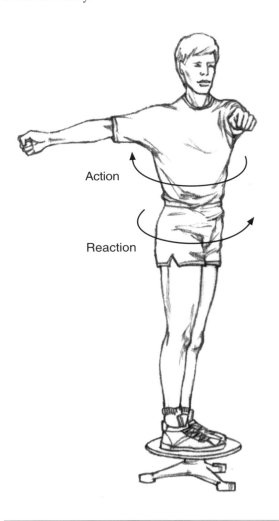

Action

Reaction

Fig. 2.8. Action and reaction demonstrated on a turntable.

Force

Whenever an athlete performs a sport skill, the athlete primarily produces internal force within the body by contracting the muscles. The muscles pull on tendons and the tendons on the bones. The force produced by the athlete then competes against the external forces produced by gravity, ground reaction force, friction, air resistance, and in many sports, the contact forces provided by opposing players.

What exactly do we mean by force? You cannot actually see a force, but you can see and experience its effects. A **force** is a push or a pull that changes or tends to change the state of motion of an athlete or an object. Here's an example that will explain what we mean by "tends to."

Imagine a weight lifter attempting to lift a barbell from the floor. The athlete reaches down and pulls on the bar. If the athlete pulls hard enough and applies sufficient force, the barbell is hoisted upward. But what happens if the athlete doesn't apply enough force to move the barbell? In this situation you could say there is a tendency for the athlete to set the barbell in motion—it is closer to moving with the athlete pulling on it than if the athlete didn't pull on it at all.

If another athlete runs onto the lifting platform and adds his force to that of the original lifter, maybe their combined force is sufficient to move the barbell off the ground. The tendency toward movement caused by the first athlete is turned into action by help from the second. The barbell moves. The force of one athlete has been added to that of the other. In this scenario you must assume that both athletes pull in the same direction. A totally different effect occurs if the second athlete pulls the barbell sideways rather than upward.

Force Vectors

In the weight-lifting scenario we imagined that two lifters combined their muscular force to lift a barbell in a vertical direction. The combination of their forces totaled a certain amount and was aimed in a particular direction. When the *direction* and *amount* of the applied force are known, the combination of these two items is called a force vector. The term *vector* simply means a quantity that has direction. In the case of the weight lifters a certain amount of force is vectored in a vertical direction.

In mechanics, force vectors are often represented diagrammatically by arrows. The head of the arrow indicates in what direction the force is acting, and the length of the arrow is scaled to appropriately represent the amount of force being applied.

In the weight-lifting situation in which one athlete lifts vertically and the other pulls the bar horizontally, the result is that they pull the barbell partially upward and partially to the side. Depending on the amount of force applied by each athlete, the barbell moves (or vectors) in a direction which is called a **resultant force vector**. The resultant force vector in this situation is the equivalent of two forces that simultaneously pull the barbell in different directions. A rough representation of what occurs can be diagrammed by using a "parallelogram of forces." One arrow (*a*) is drawn with its length and direction representing the force applied by the athlete who lifts vertically. A second arrow (*b*) is drawn to represent the force applied by the athlete who pulls the barbell horizontally. A parallelogram (opposite sides and angles equal) is drawn. The diagonal (*c*) represents the resultant force vector. This arrow and its length indicate the resultant force and the direction that the two athletes pull the barbell (see Figure 2.9).

When an athlete performs a sport skill, several forces usually act at the same time. Let's look at these forces at work in the shot put event. Think of elite athletes putting a shot at a release angle of about 42 degrees to the horizontal. To get the shot moving upward, the athletes must apply force in that direction. So the athletes apply some (but not all) of their force in a vertical direction. To get the shot moving horizontally, they apply force in that direction as well. The combination of horizontal and vertical forces gives the shot its 42-degree **trajectory**.

Obviously the shot-putters are not going to apply all of their force in just a vertical or horizontal direction. If the athletes were foolish enough to put all their force in a vertical direction, the shot would go straight up and straight down! This is hardly the right thing to do in a competition that gives the prize to the athlete who achieves the greatest horizontal distance! On the other hand, if all of the throwers' force is directed

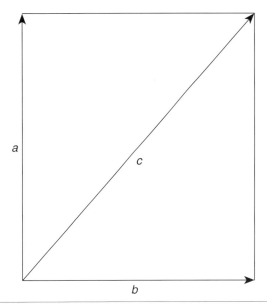

Fig. 2.9. A parallelogram of forces in weight-lifting scenario. Arrow *a* shows the force applied vertically to the barbell; arrow *b* shows the force applied horizontally to the barbell; arrow *c* shows the resultant force vector.

horizontally, the shot will hit the ground long before it has time to cover the optimal distance. So a trajectory angle is used that is partway between horizontal and vertical. For elite shot-putters who release the shot 7 ft or more above ground level, this is usually between 35 to 42 degrees.

During flight the earth's gravitational force pulls the shot directly downward (perpendicularly). So gravity fights the vertical force vector that the athletes have applied to the shot. Gravity is not interested in the horizontal force vector. In addition to the force of gravity, air resistance provides a very small force that battles the forward motion of the shot. The result of this war of forces determines the distance that the shot travels (see Figure 2.10).

There are many examples in sport of athletes combining forces to produce a desired result. Top-class defenders in soccer know from experience how long it takes for a soccer ball to travel a particular distance. They assess the velocity of the forwards on their team as they sprint into open field positions. When the defenders make a downfield pass, they consider (a) the velocity (i.e., speed and direction) that they must give to the ball and (b) the velocity of the forward sprinting to receive the pass. If a defender kicks the ball with the correct amount of force and gives it the

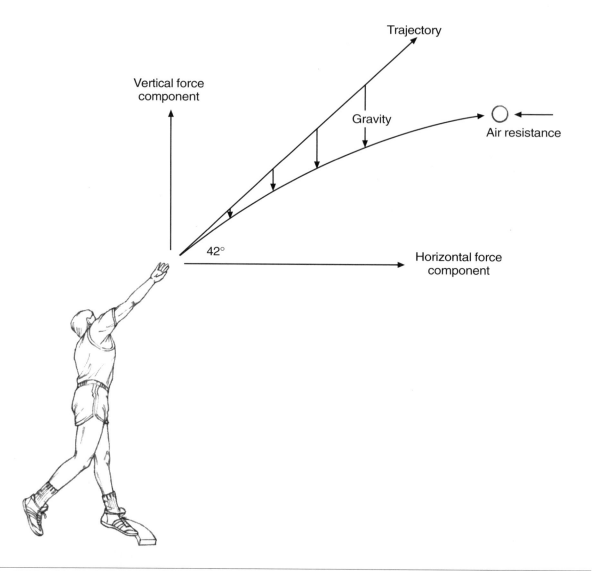

Fig. 2.10. Forces influencing the trajectory of a shot in the shot put event.

right trajetory, the ball drops at the feet of a forward who is running flat out. The same principles apply to a quarterback who wants to hit a receiver cutting across the field, or a basketball player attempting to hit a teammate who has broken away from defenders. In all cases, the passers perform a mental vector analysis to make sure that the ball arrives at a particular spot at the same time as their teammate.

An Athlete's Movement

An athlete can move in three different ways. The athlete's movement can be linear (i.e., in a straight line), angular (i.e., in a circular or rotary fashion), or a mix of linear and angular motion called "general motion."

In sport, a mix of linear and angular movement most commonly occurs, with angular movement playing the dominant role. This is because most of an athlete's movements result from the swinging, turning action of the limbs as they rotate around the joints.

Linear Motion

Linear motion, which is also called **translation**, describes a situation in which all parts of an object move the same distance, in the same direction, and in the same time. As you can imagine, this rarely occurs in an athlete, because some parts of an athlete's body can be moving while others are not. But examples do exist. A skater holding a static position and gliding in a straight line is "translating." A speed skier holding a crouched aerodynamic position and accelerating down the run is another example of linear motion.

Angular Motion

Angular motion is given many names. Coaches talk of athletes rotating, spinning, swinging, circling, turning, rolling, pirouetting, somersaulting, and twisting. All of these terms indicate that an object or an athlete is turning through an angle, or number of degrees. In sports like gymnastics, diving, and figure skating, routines include half turns (180 degrees), and full turns or "revs" (i.e., revolutions), which are 360 degrees.

To produce angular motion, movement has to occur around an axis. You can think of an axis like the axle of a wheel or the hinge on a door. An athlete's body has many joints and they all act as axes. The most visible rotary motion occurs in the arms and legs. The upper arm rotates around the shoulder joint, the lower arm around the el-bow joint, and the hand around the wrist. The hip joint acts as an axis for the leg, the knee for the lower leg, and the ankle for the foot. Movement then depends on the rotary motion of each segment (e.g., foot, shank, and thigh) of an athlete's limbs as they move around the joints.

General Motion

If you watch an athlete in a wheelchair race you will notice the swinging (angular) motion of the athlete's arms as they spin the wheels of the wheelchair. The rotary (angular) motion of the wheels carries both athlete and chair along the track. Down the straightaway the athlete and chair can be moving in a straight line. At the same time, the wheels exhibit angular motion (see Figure 2.11). This combination of angular and linear motion is known as general motion.

General motion can easily be seen in an event like sprinting. In a 100m dash athletes attempt to get from the start to the finish as quickly as possible. Even though the athletes know that the shortest distance between the start and the finish is a straight line and is best satisfied by linear motion, it is impossible to sprint in this fashion. If you watch any sprinter, you'll see a rise and

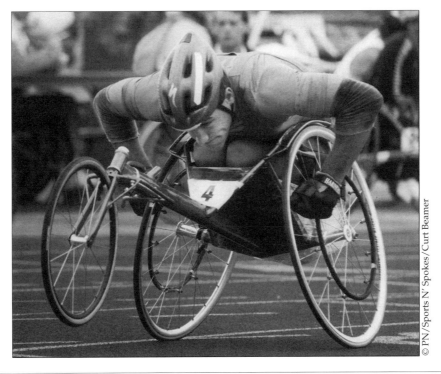

Fig. 2.11. A wheelchair athlete exhibits a combination of angular and linear motion.

fall of the athlete's body from one stride to the next. Some movement will be linear, but the greater part will be angular. In total, an athlete's sprinting action is best described as general motion.

Projectiles

In sport there are many events in which athletes and objects are projected (or propelled) into the air. The **projectiles** can be golf balls, basketballs, javelins, or, in jumping events, gymnastics, and diving, the athletes themselves. These sports all require an athlete to manipulate, control, or assess the flight path that occurs. For example, a high jumper aims for height, distance, and rotation so that she can successfully clear the bar. An archer angles the bow and pulls the string back the correct distance so that the arrow flies to the bull's-eye. A diver looks for a flight path at takeoff that gives her adequate time in the air to perform the required twists and somersaults and line up for a splashless entry. A goalkeeper in soccer assesses the velocity and flight of the ball to make a successful save. A tennis player tries to hit the ball so that it not only clears the net but also lands in the court and, equally important, beats the opponent!

In sport events that incorporate flight several factors influence the character of the flight path: trajectory and the angle, velocity, and height of the release.

Trajectory

Suppose you got rid of gravity and air resistance, and you had a pitcher throw a baseball at an angle of 35 degrees above the horizontal. Without gravity and air resistance, the baseball would fly indefinitely at a 35-degree trajectory at the velocity that the pitcher released it.

In reality, we all know that gravity pulls the baseball toward the earth. Without considering the effects that spin causes, air resistance counteracts the forward motion of the ball as it rises and falls in the air. Gravity and air resistance change the flight path of the baseball from a straight-line trajectory set at 35 degrees, to a curved flight path

in which the ball rises to a certain point and then arcs back toward the earth's surface.

Because the ball is constantly pulled toward the earth, gravity battles the rise of the ball (i.e., its vertical component) so that after a certain time it rises no more and begins its fall to the earth. The horizontal distance (or range) that the baseball travels during its flight depends on the combination of three factors.

- The angle of release (i.e., trajectory angle)
- The velocity of the baseball at the moment of release
- The height at which the baseball is released (see Figure 2.12)

All three of these factors can be varied considerably. When you add the effect of gravity, variations in air resistance, and spin imparted by the pitcher, the flight path of a baseball can resemble a limitless number of shapes. Let's look at each of the three components listed above.

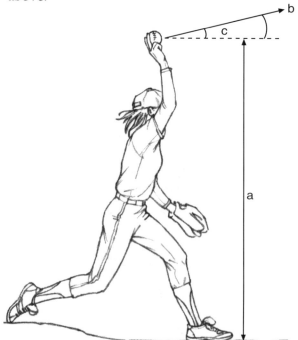

Fig. 2.12. A baseball pitcher delivers the ball at a particular height (a) and gives the ball a particular velocity (b) and angle of release (c).
Reprinted from Hall 1995.

Angle of Release

When a pitcher hurls a baseball, the shape of the ball's flight path is dependent on the angle at which the athlete releases the ball. The velocity with which the athlete throws the ball then determines the size of the flight path. So the ball's flight path can be of a different shape, and each shape can vary in size.

If you forget for a moment about air resistance, the shape of the ball's flight path tends to be one of three types.

1. If the pitcher hurls the baseball straight up, the ball goes directly upward and is pulled straight down again by gravity. The flight path is a straight line. Gravity decelerates the ball on the way up, and accelerates the ball on the way down.

2. If the pitcher hurls the ball at an angle between vertical and horizontal, an angle of release that is above 45 degrees (i.e., closer to the vertical) gives the ball a trajectory in which height dominates over distance.

3. If the pitcher hurls the ball at an angle below 45 degrees (i.e., closer to the horizontal), the flight path is long and low. The flight path has hardly any height at all. Distance dominates over height.

In reality, air resistance coupled with the shape and motion (e.g., spin) of the object causes anything but a regular-shaped flight path to occur. Think of how pitchers manipulate the flight path of a baseball and how spin, angle of release, and wind direction will alter the flight of a discus!

Velocity of Release

What happens if an object's velocity of release is varied? In this situation, if the pitcher hurls a ball straight up, an increase in the velocity of release is obviously going to make the ball go higher. The **apex** of the flight path (the highest point) is raised as the velocity of release is increased. It's the same in a vertical jump. The faster the takeoff velocity, the higher an athlete rises.

When the pitcher hurls a ball at an angle that is between vertical and horizontal, any increase in the release velocity of the ball not only increases the height of the ball, but also how far it travels.

Height of Release

The third important factor that influences the flight path of a ball is the height of release relative to the height of the surface on which it lands. Shot-putters are giant athletes who release the shot well above shoulder level, with the shot then landing at ground level. A discus thrower releases the discus at a slightly lower level than the shot-putter. Some athletes are taller than others so their body type can increase the height of release.

If it were possible for shot-putters to release a shot at ground level and the ground was perfectly horizontal, then 45 degrees would be the best release angle for the greatest distance. In this situation the athlete puts equal amounts of force in a vertical and horizontal direction. The vertical component is used to battle the downward pull of gravity. However, when an athlete releases a shot above ground level, as all shot-putters do, then to get the greatest distance, the athlete must lower the trajectory angle and release the shot at an angle that is slightly less than 45 degrees. Elite athletes release the shot at an angle that ranges from 35 to 42 degrees (see Figure 2.10). This is a large trajectory angle if you compare it with the angle used by ski jumpers when they take off. (In this situation think of the takeoff of the ski jumper in the same manner as the release of the shot. The ski jumper is a projectile just like the shot. Both fly through the air and both athlete and shot are projected for maximum distance). Ski jumpers take off from a ramp that is a long way above where they land. So they thrust themselves off at an angle that is almost horizontal. Surprisingly, ski jumpers fall down the curve of the ski jump. They hardly go upward at all!

Because long jumpers take off from ground level and want to travel as far as possible, you might guess that the takeoff angle of a long jumper would be 45 degrees. But this doesn't happen in reality. Long jumpers actually take off at an angle between 20 to 22 degrees (see Figure 2.13), and it's slightly less than this for triple jumpers. Both types of jumpers would be forced to cut their velocity down the run-up to take off at an angle of 45 degrees. No long jumper wants to do this because a reduction in run-up velocity drastically reduces the distance they travel in flight and the distance that they jump. So long jumpers compromise between velocity at takeoff and takeoff angle. Velocity is the more important factor. The result is that the takeoff angle is reduced from 45 degrees to 20 to 22 degrees.

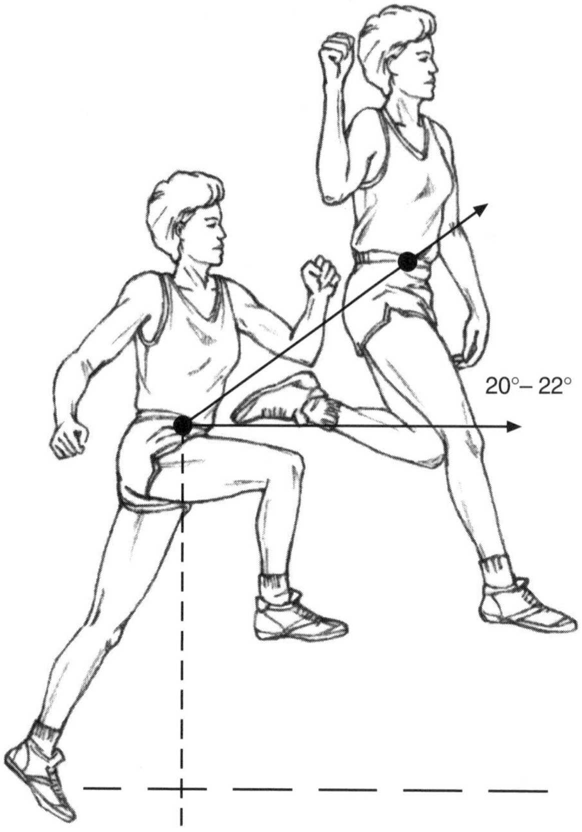

It is important for a coach to realize that velocity, height, and angle of takeoff (or release) are intrinsically tied together. Altering one component inevitably causes changes in the others. You must also consider aerodynamic and environmental factors. The javelin and discus, for example, are very much affected by the way the wind is blowing. Head winds approaching from a favorable angle and blowing at an optimal velocity (about 15-20 mph for the discus) can dramatically increase the distance that the athlete throws. With a head wind the thrower reduces not only the angle of release, but also lowers the leading edge of the discus. If the discus is tilted up too much it stalls in flight and the distance is dramatically reduced. In chapter 6 you'll read more about aerodynamic factors and how they affect the flight of discuses, javelins, baseballs, and athletes like ski jumpers.

Fig. 2.13.   Takeoff angle in the long jump.
Adapted from Kreighbaum and Barthels 1990.

SUMMARY

1. An athlete's body weight results from both the earth's gravitational pull on the athlete's body and the pull of the athlete's body on the earth. The earth's gravitational pull varies according to location.

2. All objects that have substance have mass. An athlete's body has mass, which is commonly termed body mass.

3. Mass is synonymous with inertia: the more mass, the more inertia.

4. Inertia is characterized by resistance and persistence. All objects resist movement because of their inertia. Once movement is initiated, an object's mass (and inertia) is expressed by a tendency to continue moving at a uniform speed in a straight line. This would occur if forces such as gravity, air resistance, and friction did not intervene. Massive athletes require the application of great force to get moving and the application of great force to stop or change their direction.

5. Speed is a scalar measure indicating how fast an object is traveling at a particular instant in time. An athlete who runs a 100 m in 10 sec has an average speed of 10 m/sec. Average speed does not tell us the athlete's top speed.

6. Acceleration and deceleration refer to the rate that speed changes. An athlete who increases speed at 5 ft/sec for every second in the sprint is accelerating at 5 ft/sec/sec,

or 5 ft/sec². Acceleration and deceleration are indicated with one distance unit (i.e., 5 ft) and two time units (i.e., sec/sec).

7. Velocity indicates both speed and direction.

8. The earth's gravitational acceleration is approximately 32 ft/sec² (9.8 m/sec² in the metric system). Slight variations in gravitational acceleration occur relative to location on the earth's surface.

9. The center of gravity is where the earth's gravitational pull is concentrated in an athlete's body. Changes in body position and the density of body parts shift an athlete's center of gravity.

10. Density refers to the amount of substance (or mass) contained in a particular space. Bones and muscles are more dense than body fat.

11. An athlete standing on the surface of the earth is pulled by gravity toward the earth's core. The earth reacts against the downward force exerted by the athlete by pushing upward with an equal and opposing force. This is called the earth's reaction force (or the ground reaction force).

12. Force is a push or pull that changes, or tends to change, the state of motion of an object. Athletes primarily use muscle contractions to apply force. Among the external forces affecting an athlete are gravity, air resistance, friction, the earth's reaction force, and forces applied by objects and opponents.

13. Athletic skills are made of a mix of angular (rotational) and linear (translational or straight-line) movement. This mix of movement is called "general motion." Because bones rotate at the joints, movements performed by athletes in sport skills are predominantly rotational.

14. In many sports, objects or athletes are projected or propelled into the air. Their trajectories depend on their velocity, height, and angle of release. The forces exerted by gravity and air resistance help determine the resulting flight path.

15. With no air resistance, a trajectory angle of 45° produces the greatest distance for objects projected from ground level on a horizontal surface. When the object is projected from above ground level, an angle less than 45° produces the greatest distance.

REVIEW QUESTIONS

1. Is it possible for an athlete with no change in body mass to weigh a certain amount at one place on the earth's surface and a different amount at another place?

2. A shot putter carrying a shot has it slip out of her hand and fall toward the earth. If action equals reaction, then the earth pulls on the shot with the same force that the shot pulls on the earth. If this is the case, why does the shot accelerate toward the earth?

3. The acceleration of gravity is 32 ft/sec² (i.e., 32 ft/sec/sec), or 9.8 m/sec² in the metric system. Why do we use one distance unit (i.e., 32 ft) and two time units (i.e., sec/sec) when we refer to gravity's acceleration?

4. What happens in a mechanical sense when a slalom skier weights and unweights her skis? Why does a skier carry out this maneuver?

5. What reasons relating to inertia did the text cite for elite squash and badminton players being lean and lightweight?

6. Explain how a quarterback can make a mental "vector analysis" to assure that a football arrives at a particular spot at the same time as the receiver cutting across the field.

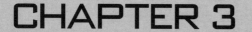

CHAPTER 3

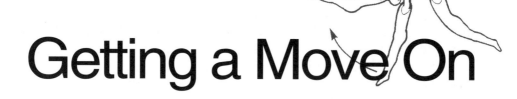

Getting a Move On

When you finish reading this chapter, you should be able to explain

- the factors that influence an object's or an athlete's acceleration;

- what is meant by impulse, and how impulse relates to acceleration and deceleration;

- how an athlete's actions cause reactions that are equal and opposite;

- what is meant by momentum, and how objects or athletes gain or lose momentum;

- the mechanical definition of work;

- the difference between power and strength;

- the relationship and differences between kinetic, potential, and strain energy;

- the factors that influence the rebound of balls; and

- the factors that control friction as objects slide or roll across contacting surfaces.

This chapter gets us involved with athletes and objects in motion. That's why we've titled it "Getting a Move On." The mechanical principles that we discuss in this chapter build on those that we've talked about in chapter 2. As you develop your knowledge about mechanics, you'll notice how all these principles tie in to one another. Equally important, you'll see that every action your athletes make in a sport skill will involve several mechanical principles at the same time. Good technique in sport is based upon making the best use of all these mechanical principles. So let's get a move on by checking out what happens when athletes apply force with their muscles and put themselves in motion.

Forces at Work in a Sprint Start

Imagine an elite sprinter in a set position. The gun goes off and the sprinter drives out of the blocks. In this situation the sprinter applies force by extending his legs against the blocks. The blocks, of course, are attached to the earth. The force (i.e., the push) that the sprinter applies against the blocks is the action. The reaction (the push back) comes from the earth pushing equally and in the opposite direction through the blocks against the sprinter (see Figure 3.1). This situation repeats the action and reaction situations that we discussed in chapter 2 when skiers weighted and unweighted their skis, and the long jumper landed in the pit with the earth pushing back equally and in the opposite direction against the jumper.

The force produced by the sprinter's muscles overcomes the athlete's inertia and the sprinter begins to accelerate. If gravity didn't exist and there was no air resistance, the sprinter's legs extending against the blocks would cause the sprinter to travel along the same path indefinitely. This is an expression of inertia. When the sprinter's body mass is moving, it wants to continue moving indefinitely in the direction that the force propels it. Gravity, friction, and air resistance put the brakes to this endless motion.

The acceleration of any sprinter's body mass is proportional to how much force the athlete applies and the time frame during which this force is applied, and is inversely proportional to how massive the athlete is. This means that if two sprinters apply the same muscular force to their bodies for the same amount of time, the more massive of the two athletes accelerates less. Likewise, if two sprinters have the same mass and apply force for the same amount of time, the athlete who applies more force will accelerate more.

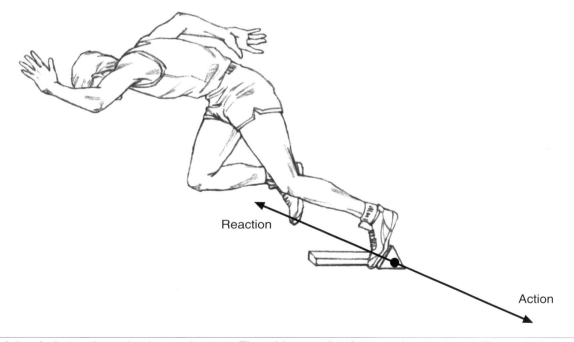

Reaction

Action

Fig. 3.1.   Action and reaction in a sprint start. The athlete applies force against the block. The earth (via the block) applies an equal and opposite force against the athlete.

By extending his legs powerfully in a sprint start, a sprinter pushes against his body mass and against the mass of the earth via the blocks. The athlete moves one direction and the earth moves an immeasurably small and negligible amount in the opposing direction. The earth and the athlete move in opposite directions relative to the size of their mass.

You can picture the relationship between the sprinter and the earth by squashing a spring between a 16 lb shot and a table tennis ball. The shot is the earth, the spring is the athlete's muscles, and the table tennis ball is the athlete. If you suddenly let go of the shot and the table tennis ball at the same time, the spring expands. The table tennis ball accelerates in one direction and the shot possibly rolls a short distance in the opposing direction. Now that you've got the idea, increase the size of the table tennis ball so it's equal to the sprinter and increase the size of the shot so it's equal to the earth. Do you see why the sprinter moves in one direction relative to his mass and the earth moves an immeasurable amount in the opposing direction relative to the earth's mass? It's easy to see why the sprinter does most of the moving!

Momentum

An athlete who is moving is an example of mass on the move. Because the athlete's body mass is moving, we say that the athlete has a certain amount of momentum. **Momentum** describes the quantity of motion that occurs. How much momentum an athlete possesses depends on how massive the athlete is and how fast the athlete is moving. Increase the athlete's mass, velocity, or both, and in each situation you increase the athlete's momentum.

Sport commentators frequently talk of a team gaining momentum, and by this they mean that one team is starting to dominate over the other. Even politicians talk of their campaigns gathering momentum. In mechanical terms momentum has a different meaning. It always takes into consideration both the velocity and the mass of an athlete or a moving object. A huge, massive athlete sprinting at the same velocity as an athlete with less body mass has more momentum. Likewise an athlete with minimal body mass

sprinting at phenomenal velocity can have more momentum than an athlete who is more massive.

To make up for a tremendous difference in mass, athletes with little body mass have to sprint at phenomenal velocity to match the momentum of a more massive athlete. As an example, if a 300 lb lineman ambled through 100 m in 20 sec, a 150 lb running back would have to flash through the same distance in 10 sec to produce the same momentum.

Momentum occurs any time an athlete or an object moves, and it plays a particularly important role in sports that have collisions and **impacts**. An easy way to think of momentum is to see it as a weapon that an athlete can use to cause an effect on another object or an opponent. A puck hit with immense velocity by a hockey player can have enough momentum to knock a goalie backward. Even though the puck is light and has little mass, some of the players in the National Hockey League hit it at tremendous velocity. When the puck hits the goalie, both puck and goalie (plus pads, mask, skates, and stick) for an instant become a combined mass. The puck slows and loses some of its momentum. It keeps a little momentum but most of it is given to the goalie, who, because he is knocked backward, gains momentum in that direction. A similar example occurs when a tennis ball is served at such velocity that it knocks the opponent's racquet backward.

Ice hockey players skate at tremendous velocities and generate great momentum. They demonstrate this in the bone-rattling checks that characterize their sport. Offensive and defensive linemen in the National Football League with their immense size and great acceleration over 40 yd also generate tremendous momentum. Like the ice hockey player, the lineman who has the most momentum at impact is likely to dominate in a collision with another player.

We have seen that if you increase either the velocity or the mass of an object or an athlete, momentum increases as well. In sport the best way for an athlete to increase mass is to put on quality muscle mass rather than fat. The extra muscle mass then provides the power to help the athlete move faster and maneuver more efficiently.

It is important to remember that not all sports situations require maximum momentum. Many skills require momentum to be carefully controlled. For example, a punter is often required to make the ball go out of bounds as close to the end zone as possible. The momentum given to the ball has to be exact so it travels a precise distance. This means that the momentum of the punter's leg kicking the ball has to be the right amount as well. Similarly, an outside shooter who fires at the basket from 3-point range aims to put the basketball through the hoop and not have it ricochet haphazardly out to midcourt. The momentum given to the ball must be exact.

Impulse

Muscular force has to be produced when an athlete wants to get moving or to accelerate an object and give it momentum. The force that the athlete applies always takes time. When an athlete applies a certain amount of force to an object over a certain time, we say that the athlete has applied an **impulse** to the object. Of course, an athlete can also apply an impulse to her own body, or to another athlete.

How force and time are combined depends on the physical capabilities of the athlete. An athlete who is strong and flexible can apply more force over a greater range (i.e., time frame) than an athlete who is weaker and less flexible. Equally important, the combination of force and time depends on the needs of the skill. Some skills require tremendous force to be applied in a short time frame. Other skills require a lesser force to be applied over a large time frame. The variations in force and time are limitless. Let's look at some examples and see how the requirements of sport skills vary the demand for force and the time of its application.

Impulse in a Karate Blow

One of the most amazing feats performed by an expert in karate is to break a block of concrete with a blow from the hand. The athlete's hand applies tremendous force to the block of concrete in a very small time frame. This feat is all the more amazing when you consider it in the light of the law of action and reaction, because what the athlete does to the concrete is done back to the athlete's hand. Surely the reaction of the concrete hitting back at the athlete would break every bone

in the athlete's hand! Sport scientists have studied this situation and have given us reasons why karate experts don't end up with their hands in casts! Blanding and Monteleone (1992) tell us, "Although it may seem that such forces should smash a hand to pieces, bones can resist 40 times more stress, or force per unit area, than concrete. Add to this the fact that the hand is not a single bone but a network of bones connected by an elastic material, and a trained hand can actually withstand forces greater than 5,000 pounds."

The impulse applied by the karate expert compresses the upper surface of the concrete and pulls the lower surfaces apart where the block is supported. Cracks appear on the lower surface and the concrete is broken in half. Beginning karate enthusiasts usually practice on even-grained dry wood and not on green lumber, which would flex rather than break! To destroy a concrete block takes years of practice before the athlete develops the proper body position and hand velocity.

Impulse in a Javelin Throw

A javelin throw differs from a karate blow because the javelin requires a different kind of impulse. Here you have tremendous force applied over a much longer time frame. Great strength and flexibility are required in this event. An expert javelin thrower accelerates the javelin by pulling it from way behind the body and releasing it far out in front. Long arms are beneficial as is a backward lean when entering the throwing position. In this way the athlete applies force over a huge distance (and a long time period) to the javelin. To a spectator it may not seem that the athlete is accelerating the javelin for very long because a good javelin throw seems to happen so quickly. But when an elite thrower is compared with a novice, the distinction between the two athletes is easy to see, even to a person who is not familiar with the event. To start with, the elite thrower is much stronger and applies more force to the javelin. Second, greater flexibility and careful technical training allow the elite athlete to accelerate the javelin over a greater distance. Consequently, more force is applied over a longer time frame to the javelin. The result is that the impulse applied to the javelin is greater and it moves at a tremendous velocity when it is released (see Figure 3.2).

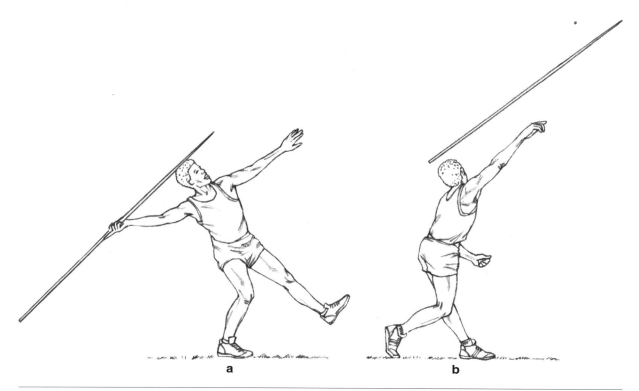

Fig. 3.2. Impulse in a javelin throw. Elite athletes are able to apply force over a long time frame by (a) leaning back and pulling the javelin from behind the body and (b) releasing it far out in front.

Impulse at Takeoff in the High Jump

High jump is similar to javelin in that both events require the athlete to generate tremendous release velocity. In high jump, the athlete is a projectile propelled upward into the air by muscular force. In the javelin throw, the javelin is a projectile hurled by the thrower. Because the high jumper wants to go as high as possible, you might think it would be a good idea at takeoff to apply as much force as possible over the largest available time frame. So why not have the athlete start the upward thrust at takeoff from a full squat position and keep thrusting until the jumping leg is fully extended? Surely starting from a full squat maximizes the time that force is applied by the leg muscles. Unfortunately this is not the case. In a full squat an athlete cannot develop maximum force because the leg muscles are in a poor posi-

Rules Limit High Jumpers

The rules of high jump specify that competitors must take off from one foot. If a two-footed takeoff were allowed, the world record of just over 8 ft would surely be held by a gymnast using a high speed run-up, a round off, several back handsprings, and a triple back somersault to cross the bar. On the second of the three somersaults today's elite gymnasts reach heights of 9 and 10 ft. Forty years ago, before gymnasts had mastered triple somersaults, they had already back-somersaulted over a bar set at 7 ft 6 in.

tion to drive the athlete upward. What you'll find instead is that all great high jumpers apply tremendous force for a shorter time and start their upward thrust from a position that resembles a 1/4 squat. If high jumpers cannot use a fully flexed position, is there any other way they can extend the time frame over which they apply force? Yes. Just like an elite javelin thrower, all great jumpers lean backward as they plant the jumping foot prior to takeoff. Straightening from the backward lean allows the athlete to spend more time applying force to the ground, which in reaction, thrusts the athlete upward (see Figure 3.3). The same technique is used by volleyball players when they jump to spike and block, by soccer players when they jump to head the ball, and by basketball players when they leap to block or perform a layup. The use of a backward lean before takeoff helps all athletes to get higher in the air.

Impulse and Cadence in Sprinting, Speed Skating, and Rowing

Sprinting, speed skating, and rowing are similar in that athletes repeat a certain skill in a cyclic fashion throughout the race. They are not like the high jump in which the athlete gets a rest after a jump, or the volleyball spike in which another skill like blocking or digging can occur immediately after the spike. Elite sprinters repeat their sprinting action for approximately 10 sec in a 100m sprint. Rowers repetitively pull on the oars for just under 6 min in an eights competition. Throughout the race these athletes change the amount and the time frame that they apply force with their muscles. At the start rowing eights use more strokes per minute when they accelerate than they do farther down the course. Each pull on the oar is quick, powerful, but over a short range or distance. Likewise, sprinters and speed

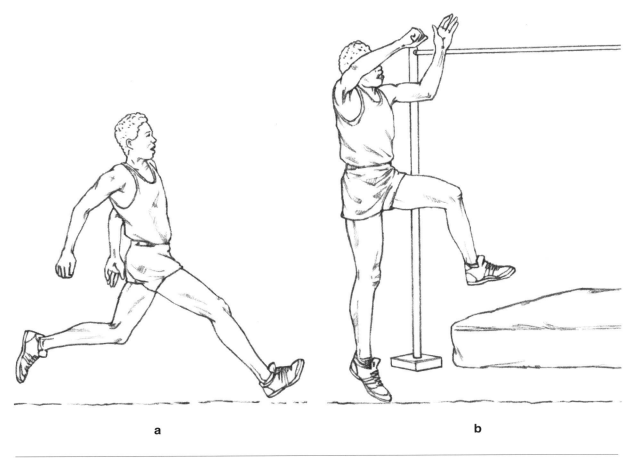

a   b

Fig. 3.3.   Impulse in a flop high jump takeoff. Elite high jumpers lean back prior to take-off (a), which allows them to spend more time applying force to the earth (b). The earth, in reaction, thrusts the athlete upward.

skaters use short, quick, choppy strides as they accelerate from the start. Once moving at high velocity they reduce their stride rate but each stride is longer. Why? The answer is that great force applied quickly and repeatedly over a short distance, or a short range of motion, is the most efficient way of overcoming inertia. It's the best way for a rowing eight or a sprinter to accelerate and get up to top velocity. Unfortunately, a high stroke or stride rate burns up a lot of energy, and although efficient when accelerating, it is inefficient once moving at high velocity. At this velocity, sprinters and speed skaters reduce their stride or rate and extend more fully with each leg thrust. Rowers pull over a larger distance with each stroke using a greater range of motion. So even though the stride rate and stroke rate are reduced, great force is now applied over an increased range of motion at a lower cadence. This "change-down" helps the athletes to maintain their velocity without "running out of gas."

Using Impulse to Slow Down and Stop

Let's look at impulse in a different light. In this section you'll see how impulse is used to slow down and stop an object. Here's an example. A field hockey player hits a ball and it rolls across the turf. Friction with the turf coupled with a small amount of air resistance slowly brings the ball to a halt. The small forces of friction and air resistance are applied to the ball over a long time (and distance), and the result is that they progressively reduce the momentum of the ball to zero. At any instant in time the force applied to the ball is small, but it is applied progressively over a long time.

Compare the forces working on the field hockey ball to those working on a basketball player who leaps for a slam dunk and afterward lands stiff legged on the floor. The player's mass dropping from a height slams into the floor and comes to a halt in an instant. The reaction force of the floor (i.e., the earth) hits back at the athlete with the same force that the athlete hits the floor. Unfortunately the time during which the athlete's body must absorb these forces is extremely small. So the shock and stress on the athlete's body are phenomenal. What do most athletes do naturally to counteract this? They flex at the ankles, knees, and hips. When you coach, you tell your athlete

to "bend your legs as you land!" (Most athletes perform this action naturally!) In a mechanical sense, your coaching advice tells the athlete to extend the time during which the athlete's body receives and absorbs the forces applied by the ground. At any instant over this longer time frame, the force applied to the athlete's body will be less.

In sport you'll find situations in which it's difficult to extend the time to soften the impact. A first baseman reaching to catch a ball will be fully extended and cannot always draw the hand to extend the time of contact with the ball. But the glove helps. Its padding extends the time of contact, and you'll see later that its design also extends the area of contact with the ball. This feature helps to absorb the forces applied by the ball.

In addition to enlarging the time frame that force is applied to their bodies, athletes are taught to enlarge the point of impact (i.e., the place where forces are applied) to as large an area as possible. A runner's slide into home base is a good example. The slide not only gets the runner's legs below the reach of the opponent's tag, but it extends the time during which friction with the ground brings the athlete to a halt. In addition, the sliding action puts a large area of the runner's body in contact with the ground. Visualize the pain and discomfort of a runner who dives at the bag headfirst and stops in an instant on the point of his nose! Although this comical scenario seldom occurs, it illustrates a situation in which all the forces produced by the athlete are reduced to zero in an instant and in a very small and sensitive area.

There are many sports in which athletes are taught specific techniques so that they extend the area and time that forces act on their bodies. By doing this they avoid injury and reduce to comfortable levels the pressures exerted on their bodies. Ski jumpers flex their legs when they land, and this absorbs the impact forces of the landing (see Figure 3.4). Ice hockey players try to ride out the force of a check from an opponent, and athletes in judo use break-fall techniques that enlarge the area and the time frame that the force of impact with the mat (i.e., the earth) is applied to their bodies. Perhaps one of the most famous examples of this mechanical principle was Muhammad Ali's legendary "rope-a-dope" technique of rolling with the punch. As the opponent threw a punch, Muhammad Ali rolled his head and body backward. In this way the force of the opponent's punch was extended over a longer

Learning New Dives Without Pain

Divers in training now land on a bed of air bubbles. As the diver drops toward the water the coach triggers the release of pressurized air from the bottom of the diving tank. The air expands as it rises and at the surface it provides an elevated area of frothy water. It doesn't matter if athletes fail in a dive because there's a bed of watery air bubbles that cushions them as they hit the water. Divers can belly flop from the 10 m tower knowing that at 33 mph most of the sting of a poor dive has been eliminated.

time frame and so had less effect. Imagine the difference if Muhammad had stepped into a punch thrown by his opponent. The time frame of contact would have been reduced to an instant and the effect of the punch would have been much greater!

Athletes are not alone in trying to avoid injury by using special techniques when they are involved in impact situations. They get help from equipment that is designed to extend the time and enlarge the area over which external forces are applied to the athlete's body. Helmets, padding, gloves, crash pads, and air-pits do this job. The total force applied to the athlete's body may not change, but by extending the time and the area of application, the forces applied at any one instant and in any one place on the athlete's body are significantly reduced.

Work

In everyday use, "work" usually means some kind of activity not as pleasurable as "play." Working out in the weight room, even though it can be fun, gives the connotation of labor and hard work.

In mechanics, when **work** is done it means that a force has been applied against a resistance over a particular distance. In other words, work in mechanical terms = force × distance. Because distance is involved, something visible occurs and an object or an athlete moves from here to there. We've already discussed some examples of mechanical work being performed. The javelin thrower applied force to the javelin over a certain distance, and in doing this performed work

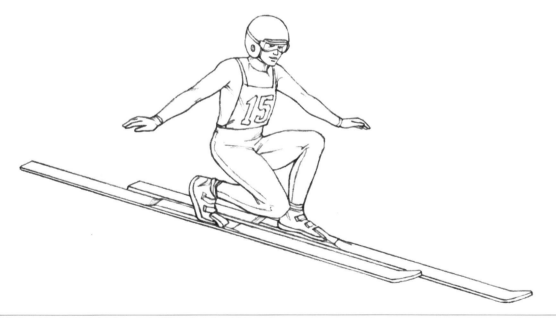

Fig. 3.4.   Reducing the impact of landing in ski jumping.

on the javelin. In our field hockey example, when the grass slowly brought the field hockey ball to a stop, the grass was progressively applying force to the ball. This is an expression of mechanical work also. In both cases, force was applied over a large distance.

In weight training, curling a dumbbell is a good example of mechanical work. The athlete applies force to the dumbbell, and as a result raises the dumbbell a certain distance. On the other hand, if a bar is fixed at chest height in a rack and an athlete presses or pulls against it for a 10 sec static contraction, no work is done in a mechanical sense because nothing moves. It doesn't matter how vigorously the athlete's muscles contract or how much physiological work is done. If nothing moves, whether it's a javelin, field hockey ball, or a dumbbell, no mechanical work is done.

Power

Power refers to the amount of mechanical work done in a particular time period. In everyday life we use **horsepower** as a measure of the power of engines such as those used in the Indy 500. One horsepower is the ability of an engine (or a human) to move 550 lb over a distance of 1 ft in 1 sec. How is power used in athletic contests? Using a weight-lifting example, imagine two athletes lifting the same weight barbell. One takes 2 sec to lift the barbell overhead, and the other takes 1 sec. They both lift the barbell the same distance. In this comparison the latter athlete is more powerful. Why? Both athletes moved the same weight over the same distance and performed similar amounts of mechanical work. But the second athlete took less time and so is considered more powerful.

Here's another example illustrating power. Let's imagine that two great athletes like Carl Lewis and Linford Christie race against each other over 100 m and both cross the line in 9.8 sec. On the day of the race, Linford is heavier and more massive than Carl. This means that Linford is more powerful because he moved more mass over the same distance (100 m) in the same time frame (9.8 sec). This description also indicates that power differs from strength because **strength** does not necessarily imply the applica-

tion of force with velocity. Perhaps on this basis, the sport of power lifting, which tends to measure strength rather than power in squats, bench press, and dead lift, should be called "strength lifting."

In most sports, power is tremendously important because a slow application of force will not get the job done. This is particularly the case in throwing and jumping events, Olympic weight lifting (i.e., the snatch and clean and jerk), and a sport like gymnastics in which skills like back and front somersaults cannot be performed slowly. Successful performance in these events demands that great force is applied very quickly!

Energy

Energy is the capacity of an athlete or an object to do work. In a mechanical sense energy can have three forms.

Kinetic Energy

This is the capacity of an object (or an athlete) to do work by virtue of being on the move. The more mass it has, and in particular, the faster it moves, the greater its capacity to do work. Any object that is moving has both momentum and **kinetic energy**.

Potential Energy

This is a form of stored energy—energy that is available and ready to be put to work. An object (or an athlete) has **potential energy** when it has height (i.e., above the earth's surface). The greater the height and weight the more potential energy.

Strain Energy

This is also a form of stored energy. Objects have **strain energy** if they have the ability to rebound or recoil after they have been squashed, pulled, twisted, or pushed out of their original (resting) shape. Obviously work has to be done to put an object into this condition and, once distorted, the ability of an object to rebound or recoil means that it can do work too. The elastic recoil of stretched muscles as athletes run, jump, and throw is also an example of strain energy at work.

Kinetic, Potential, and Strain Energy in Action

Kinetic, potential, and strain energy are all well demonstrated in the pole vault. In this event an athlete like 20 ft vaulter Sergei Bubka sprints flat out down the runway carrying the pole. The kinetic energy developed during the run-up (because the athlete's mass is in motion) is used to bend the pole, which gives it strain energy.

Bending the pole is a form of mechanical work. If the athlete runs more slowly, the pole bends less, and less strain energy is stored in it. This tells you why world-class pole-vaulters like Sergei Bubka are such superb sprinters! The faster they can run, the higher they can hold on the pole. A high handhold helps to flex a stiffer and more powerful pole. If you can bend this kind of pole, you store a tremendous amount of strain energy in it (see Figure 3.5).

During the vault, the pole straightens out, lifting the athlete up toward the bar. The strain energy stored in the pole is now converted into kinetic energy (because the athlete is propelled upward), and because the athlete is rising in the air, the potential energy of the athlete increases also. At the top of the vault the athlete rises no higher. Kinetic energy is now zero because the athlete is momentarily not moving. But the athlete is a long way above the surface of the earth and so has considerable potential energy. As the athlete accelerates toward earth, potential energy is progressively replaced by kinetic energy. By the time the athlete hits the landing pad, he is moving fastest and so has tremendous kinetic energy. The athlete's mass depresses the landing pad, making the contacting surfaces slightly warmer. The squashing of the landing pad and the heat developed are expressions of the work done by the kinetic energy of the vaulter.

There are many other examples of these three types of energy occurring in sport. Bending a bow in archery or flexing a springboard in diving are examples of work being performed on an object

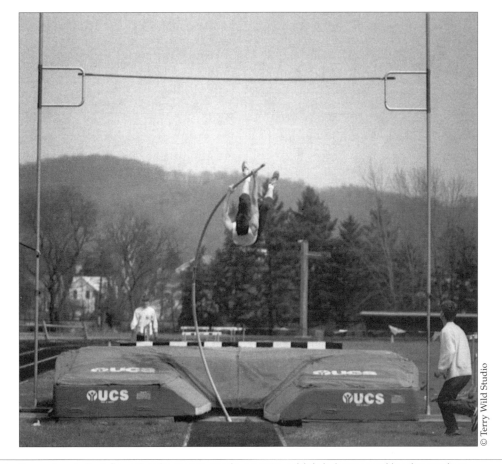

Fig. 3.5. In the pole vault, a flexed pole stores strain energy, which is later used by the vaulter.

to give it strain energy. In gymnastics, a trampolinist uses muscular force to stretch the springs of the trampoline. The stretched springs have strain energy. This energy performs work by propelling the trampolinist into the air. The trampolinist has zero kinetic energy when, for a brief instant, she is motionless at the top of her flight path. At this point her potential energy is maximal. At liftoff and when she contacts the trampoline bed again on the way down, her velocity and kinetic energy are maximal and her potential energy minimal. The kinetic energy generated during the fall toward the trampoline bed is combined with force applied by the trampolinist's muscles. Both perform work to stretch the trampoline springs once again.

How Kinetic Energy and Momentum Are Related

All objects that are on the move have both momentum and kinetic energy. Depending on how much mass they have and how fast they are moving, they have the capacity to apply force against other objects (or against themselves) over a particular distance and time frame. Let's look at how momentum and kinetic energy are related and how they differ.

The easiest way to think of kinetic energy is to regard it as the ability of a moving object to do work on whatever it contacts! The moving object can be any object you like. It can be an athlete running into an opponent, or an arrow shot by an archer and piercing a target. If the moving object has the ability to do work, then it can apply force over a particular distance to whatever it hits. The athlete drives into the opponent, the pole-vaulter compresses the landing pads a certain distance, and the arrow buries itself a certain depth in the target.

Of kinetic energy's two components (mass and velocity), velocity is particularly important, because every increase in velocity squares the amount of kinetic energy that an object possesses, whereas doubling the mass only doubles the kinetic energy. This means that if you keep the mass of a moving object the same and you double its velocity, then the object's kinetic energy is increased fourfold. With four times the kinetic energy, it's ability to do work on something it hits is increased four times as well! Take the archer's arrow as an example:

If the archer doubles the mass of the arrow and fires it at the same velocity, then the arrow sinks into the target approximately twice as deep. If the archer doubles the velocity of the arrow and keeps its mass the same, then the arrow sinks into the target approximately four times as deep! In both cases, some of the arrow's kinetic energy will be dissipated as heat, slightly warming the arrowhead and the pierced target area.

In sport whenever an athlete is on the move, the athlete has both momentum and kinetic energy. Let's consider tackling in football and see how momentum and kinetic energy are related but also different. Imagine a 300 lb lineman entering a tackle at a velocity of 4 ft/sec. At this velocity the lineman has $300 \times 4 = 1,200$ units of momentum. A 150 lb safety sprinting into a tackle at 8 ft/sec has the same amount of momentum (i.e., $150 \times 8 = 1,200$) (see Figure 3.6). If their opponents both weigh 200 lb and run at 6 ft/sec, then they will also have 1,200 units of momentum. In the tackle both the lineman and the safety are equally effective in stopping their opponents, because in each tackle 1,200 units of momentum runs into 1,200 units!

Now let's look at the kinetic energy involved in the two tackles. Because the safety sprints at 8 ft/sec, he goes into the tackle twice as fast as the lineman, who enters his tackle at 4 ft/sec. If the lineman and the safety have the same mass, the safety would have four times the kinetic energy of the lineman because he runs twice as fast. But at 150 lb he has half the mass of the 300 lb lineman. So his kinetic energy is 4 divided by 2, or twice as much as the lineman.

How is double the amount of kinetic energy expressed in the tackle? Think of the archer's arrow going into the target, or the pole-vaulter compressing the landing pads. In his tackle the safety is going to do twice as much work on his opponent as the lineman. Think of him driving himself twice as deep (just like the archer's arrow) into his opponent's body! The result of this extra ability to do work causes a lot of pain and even broken bones for both the 200 lb opponent and for the 150 lb safety!

The lesson to be learned from these examples is that when anything moves at high velocity it has a tremendous capacity to apply force over a particular distance. This capacity can often be expressed as damage when there's a collision. In

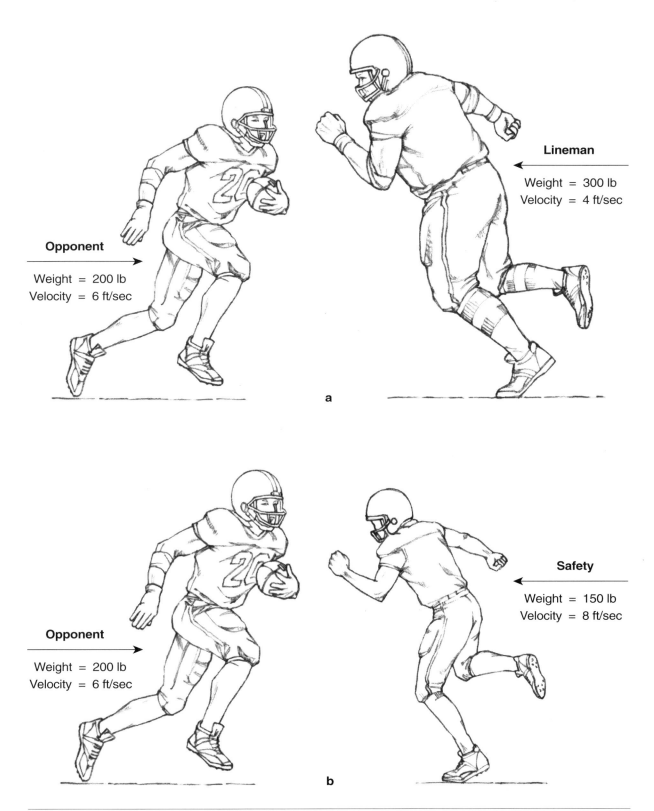

Opponent

Weight = 200 lb
Velocity = 6 ft/sec

Lineman

Weight = 300 lb
Velocity = 4 ft/sec

a

Opponent

Weight = 200 lb
Velocity = 6 ft/sec

Safety

Weight = 150 lb
Velocity = 8 ft/sec

b

Fig. 3.6. Momentum and kinetic energy in a tackle. The lineman in (a) and the safety in (b) each have 1,200 units of momentum, but the safety has twice as much kinetic energy.

car accidents, metal is bent and squashed by the kinetic energy of the moving vehicles. In sport, lightweight athletes who enter tackles at phenomenal velocity are likely to hurt not only their opponents but themselves as well.

Kinetic energy also figures prominently in baseball batting. It is well known among batters that it is better to increase the velocity of the bat rather than swing a heavier bat. Blanding and Monteleone (1992) estimate that, "For each mile an hour increase in bat speed, a batter should be able to get five extra feet out of the drive." What this tells you is that the kinetic energy generated by a lighter bat will produce more homers because it moves faster (and so does more work on the ball) than a heavier bat. Some players know this fact and have tried to reduce the weight of a bat illegally—like drilling a hole down the barrel of the bat and filling it with cork. This ploy will reduce the weight of the bat by over an ounce, but it's embarrassing when the weakened bat shatters and cork flies all over the field.

How Kinetic Energy Can Be Dissipated

Examples for safely dissipating the energy of a moving object occur throughout sport. For example, a baseball heading toward a fielder at a high velocity has plenty of kinetic energy. When the fielder catches and stops the ball, the ball does work on the fielder. The fielder can commit the error of stopping the ball with rigid hands and arms, in which case all the force of the ball is expended on the fielder over a very short distance and time frame. The fielder can also draw the arms back and recoil with the ball the instant contact is made. Of course, this is what most fielders do! In this situation the force of the ball is spread over a longer distance. It's obvious which of the two methods is less painful and less likely to cause injury.

If this example brings to mind our earlier discussion of how athletes dissipate the momentum of a moving object, that's because anything on the move has both momentum and kinetic energy. To avoid injury, an athlete's goal is to increase the area over which an impact occurs and to increase the distance and time frame that force is applied to the athlete's body.

Rebound

When bats hit balls or balls bounce off floors, a collision or impact occurs. When the objects separate, and one (or both) move away from the other, we say they have **rebounded**. What actually happens during and after the collision depends on many interacting factors. Let's look at what happens to balls when they are hit and as they bounce.

On many occasions both the ball and the object it collides with are moving (like a racquet hitting a ball). Sometimes one object can be moving and the other can be momentarily stationary (like a bowling ball hitting a pin). After the collision the bowling ball slows down slightly and loses momentum. The pin accelerates and gains momentum. In another common situation, one object (like a squash ball or basketball) is moving and then collides and rebounds from an immense stationary object like a wall or the floor.

In the examples given above, the angle that the collision occurs can vary. Both objects can hit head-on, like a basketball dropped straight down and bouncing on the floor, or they can glance off one another at an angle like a carom shot in pool, handball, or a bounce pass in basketball.

Rebound and Elastic Recoil

An important factor in determining what happens after a collision is the degree of elastic recoil that objects have. (By elastic recoil, we mean the force by which objects push back to their original shape.) Some objects have very little **elasticity** and recoil, and stick together like clay after colliding. A Hacky Sack ball has no bounce at all. Likewise an athlete who falls out of control onto the ground hardly bounces back up into the air. The human body in this condition has very little elasticity!

Golf balls, on the other hand, are well known for their elastic recoil. They are deformed (squashed out of shape) when hit by a club. Like a spring that is compressed, the ball stores strain energy, which is transformed into kinetic energy as it regains shape. The kinetic energy contributes to the velocity of the ball and in the fact that the ball is a little warmer after it has been hit. Just like the pole-vaulter's pole, strain energy produces kinetic energy, which makes a contribution toward the velocity of the golf ball as it comes off the club face. The same thing happens to a baseball when it is hit. A baseball is squashed or flattened to almost half its size when it is hit for a home run. As the ball leaves the bat, it springs back to its original shape. The energy produced by this action adds velocity to the flight of the ball. This extra energy helped great hitters like Babe Ruth and Reggie Jackson put the ball out of the park or in the upper row of the bleachers.

The elastic recoil of any object also depends on the nature of the object with which it collides. A football can rebound with considerable velocity off artificial surfaces. This differs dramatically from the rebound that occurs when the ball drops on wet, muddy turf.

Rebound and Temperature

Temperature makes a difference in the way balls rebound after a collision. Heat causes the air inside a ball to expand, and this increases the ball's ability to rebound. In squash, players spend time before a match rallying back and forth so that the ball is hot and bouncing correctly. A cold squash ball, in contrast, is a dead ball—with little or no bounce—making it much more difficult for players to return a shot. Elite A-level squash players are required to play with a ball designed to bounce very little, even when it's warmed up and the air inside it is hot. In this way the elite players are challenged according to their ability. Novices, on the other hand, use a ball designed to bounce much higher after it is warmed up. The ball's additional time in flight gives the novice players more time to get into position and make their strokes.

Angle, Velocity, and Frictional Forces in a Rebound

Many factors determine what happens to a ball after it collides with another object. In addition to those items already mentioned, the bounce or rebound of a ball depends on the angle and velocity that the ball contacts the surface, whether the ball is spinning, and finally how much friction occurs between the ball and whatever it is hitting. These factors play a big part in table tennis. In this sport the rough, spongy surface of the bat imparts tremendous spin to the ball. Even

though the ball and the table have smooth surfaces, the effect of the spinning ball hitting the table at high velocity is dramatic. The direction of rotation of a topspin makes the ball accelerate off the table at a low angle. A backspin causes the reverse to occur. Its spin is in opposition to the ball's movement. Using a backspin, an elite table tennis player can make the ball land on the opponent's side of the table and then have the ball jump back across the net!

The direction of spin plays a tremendous role in many sports. In billiards, the spin (or "English") given to the cue ball affects what happens to the ball the cue ball strikes, and to the cue ball itself afterward. Similarly, in golf, backspin applied to a golf ball by the angle or loft of the club face helps to give the ball lift and enables it to stay in the air longer. (You'll read more about lift in chapter 6.) In basketball, good shooting requires that the athlete give the ball a backspin at the instant of release. This is done by making the ball roll off the fingertips as it leaves the shooter's hand. A basketball shot with backspin that hits the rim or the backboard not only loses velocity when it hits, but the backward rotation makes it more likely to drop in the basket. Rick Barry, one of the greatest foul shooters ever to play basketball (.900 average) was well known for his underhand shooting technique. He could throw the ball with considerable backspin in this manner, and the backspin was instrumental in rotating the ball down into the basket. Of course, you still have to be accurate. Wilt Chamberlain tried copying Rick's technique without much success.

Most modern basketball players shoot fouls the same way they shoot during the game. Even though they shoot overhand, the finger flick applied at the end of their action produces backspin. The backspin then helps to sink the ball in the basket (see Figure 3.7). A topspin, on the other hand, is more likely to cause the ball to rebound back out into the court.

Rebound in Tennis

The game of tennis is in many ways more complex than table tennis because of the number of factors that affect the rebound of the ball. For example, a tennis court can be clay, grass, or a hard surface. All these surfaces have a different effect on the way the ball rebounds. Courts can be indoors or

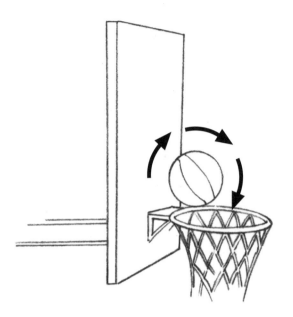

Fig. 3.7. A backspin helps to sink the ball in the basket. Adapted from Blanding and Monteleone 1992.

outdoors, and environmental conditions like temperature, humidity, and wind velocities alter play. Tennis racquets vary in size, shape, weight, and flexibility, and strings differ in type and in tension. Even the tennis ball itself changes in the way it reacts. Tennis balls bounce higher after they are warm and after some nap (fuzz) is worn off. When they have been out of their pressurized cans for a long time, the balls age and lose their bounce irrespective of how much use they've had.

These examples illustrate factors that affect the outcome of many types of impacts that occur in sport. Most athletes and coaches learn by experience and experimentation what to expect. What is important is that you stay abreast of changes that occur in equipment and playing surfaces.

These changes, which are occurring every day, always require modifications in the techniques used by your athlete.

Friction

Friction is a force that occurs when an object moves or tends to move while in contact with another object. It is present when a jogger's running shoes make contact with the road and when a bowling ball rolls down the surface of the lane. In both these examples friction occurs between two solid surfaces. However, friction also results when a ski jumper or javelin flies through air or when swimmers move through water. In these situations both the water and the air act as fluids, and they produce fluid friction; we'll examine fluid friction in chapter 6, concentrating in this chapter specifically on friction that occurs between *solid* surfaces.

The demands for friction vary dramatically from one sport to the next and from one set of environmental conditions to another. An athlete may want plenty of friction at one instant and only minimal friction at another. In cross-country skiing the correct choice of wax relative to the snow conditions allows sufficient friction for traction but not so much friction that an athlete cannot glide on the skis when necessary. In football, making sudden changes of direction depends on friction for good traction. On artificial turf friction between an athlete's shoe and the turf can sometimes be too good! During tackles the athlete's foot can get trapped in one

Technology Changes the Tennis Racquet

The sweet spot is that part of a tennis racquet that returns the ball with the greatest velocity and with the least shock and vibration to the player. Modern tennis racquets have increased in size from 75 sq in for the old wooden racquets to 95 to 100 sq in for modern composites. On wooden racquets the sweet spot was close to the base of the racquet face. Modern composite racquets have a larger sweet spot, which is higher on the racquet. In addition, modern composite racquets are stiffer so that they transfer more energy to the ball. With a higher sweet spot, the ball is hit more reliably, less shock is felt by the player, and the ball comes off the racquet faster!

position. The result frequently is torsion (i.e., twisting) injuries to the knee and ankle.

Tennis professionals, such as Pete Sampras, Steffi Graf, and Andre Agassi, compete on three different surfaces: hard courts, grass, and clay. Hard courts vary in texture, and the more grit used in the top dressing, the more friction will occur between the ball and the court surface. If you increase friction, you will slow down the ball as it rebounds off the surface. Grass provides very little friction. The short grass at Wimbledon is known as a fast surface: It benefits power players with rocket serves, like Pete Sampras. Clay is the polar opposite of grass. Rough clay courts, like those in the Roland Garros Stadium in Paris, are known as extremely slow surfaces: These surfaces reduce the effectiveness of the serve and volley game of power players who dominate on faster grass and hard courts. On clay defenders have more time to get to the ball and to counterattack. The strategy of clay court specialists, like Austria's Thomas Muster (winner of the 1995 French Open), is to hit passing shots over and past power players. Thomas Muster is king of the endurance battles that occur on clay court surfaces. In 1995 he proved his supremacy by winning 35 clay court tournaments in succession!

Types of Friction

Three types of friction occur between solid surfaces. The first is *static friction*, which exists between the contacting surfaces of two resting objects and provides the resistive force opposing the initiation of motion. The second type of friction is *sliding friction*, the resistive force that develops when two objects slide and rub against each other. The third type of friction is *rolling friction*, which produces resistive force when objects—such as balls and wheels—roll over a supporting or contacting surface. In sport sometimes all three of these frictional forces oppose the motion of a single object. For example, a field hockey ball at rest resists movement initially because of the static friction existing between the ball and the turf. Once a player hits the ball, it may simultaneously slide and roll, in which case both sliding and rolling friction resist its motion. Only rolling friction, however, remains once the ball is fully rolling and no longer sliding.

Let's examine static, sliding, and rolling fric-

tion by looking at a football player shoving a blocking sled, a common piece of equipment designed to slide on turf and provide both static and mobile (i.e., sliding) resistance against a player.

Static and Sliding Friction. The frictional force generated by a blocking sled at rest comes from static friction. If an athlete pushes against the sled with minimal effort, the sled remains motionless. In this situation the static friction is greater than the force produced by the athlete. If the athlete increases his thrust against the sled, the frictional force opposing the athlete reaches a critical level called the sled's *maximum static friction*. Should the athlete further increase the force of his push, he will overcome the sled's maximum static friction and the sled will start to slide. Static friction is now replaced by a frictional force between the base of the sled and the turf called sliding, or *kinetic*, friction. Sliding friction is always less than maximum static friction. In other words, it's easier to keep an object moving than to start it moving.

Now that we know the difference between static and sliding friction, let's look at the factors that influence the amount of static and sliding friction that can occur.

• **The force pressing the two surfaces together.** Using the blocking sled as an example, the force pressing the base of the sled to the turf is equal to the weight of the sled pushing down and the reaction of the earth pushing up. These two forces press the contacting surfaces of sled and turf together. If a coach gets on the sled, both the weight of the sled pressing downward and the reaction force of the earth pressing upward increase as well. The frictional force opposing an athlete attempting to push the sled will therefore be greater.

The importance of weight (or mass) pressing two surfaces together cannot be overemphasized. More mass means more pressure thrusting the contacting surfaces of turf and sled together. For the maximal friction, the weight of the sled plus whatever weight is added must act perpendicularly to the supporting surface. If a coach hangs on the sled with his body angled (so that he is not standing upright), only part of his weight contributes to pushing the sled down onto the turf.

• **The actual contact area between the two surfaces.** Actual is the important word here, since friction can occur only where there is contact between two surfaces. Where part of the base of the blocking sled does not contact the ground, friction cannot occur. If an athlete lifts the sled by pushing forward and upward, then no friction occurs where the sled loses contact with the ground (see Figure 3.8). Likewise, if a soccer player's studs are the only part of the boot contacting the ground, then only the surface of the studs contributes to the contacting area; the rest of the sole makes no contact and generates no friction.

Here is an example that illustrates the importance of the union between the actual contact area (i.e., the parts of the surfaces in contact) and the forces pressing the two surfaces together. Imagine two sleds that weigh the same but have bases of different sizes. An athlete pushes against one sled and then in exactly the same manner (and with the same force) against the other. The larger sled will be no more difficult to push than the smaller. Why? Because the weight of the bigger sled is spread over a bigger area and presses onto the turf proportionally less for every square inch of its base. Consequently, the same friction is produced by both sleds.

• **The nature and type of materials that are in contact.** The nature and type of materials in contact refer not only to the material on the base of the sled but also to the type of surface that the sled contacts. Imagine that the base of the sled is rough and pitted, and it is forced to slide over a muddy, sticky surface. The frictional force opposing the player would be greater with this sled than the force produced by a sled with a smooth base sliding over a hardened, level surface. The many different materials used in sport (and everyday life) all produce varying levels of friction as they contact one another. At one end of the scale, for example, consider the long steel blades of a speed skater gliding on ice: The thin film of water produced by the blade pressing on the ice produces a lubricant that reduces friction to an extremely low level. At the other end of the scale, court shoes with gum rubber soles pressing against a rubberized surface, create a tremendously high level of friction.

• **The relative motion between the two surfaces.** The relative motion between the base of the blocking sled and the ground refers to whether the athlete is applying force to *initiate* movement or whether the sled is already moving. Remember that static friction produces a higher level of resistance than sliding friction. We all have experienced the fact that it's easier to keep an object sliding than to start it sliding.

Rolling Friction. Rolling friction occurs when a round object, such as a ball or wheel, rolls across

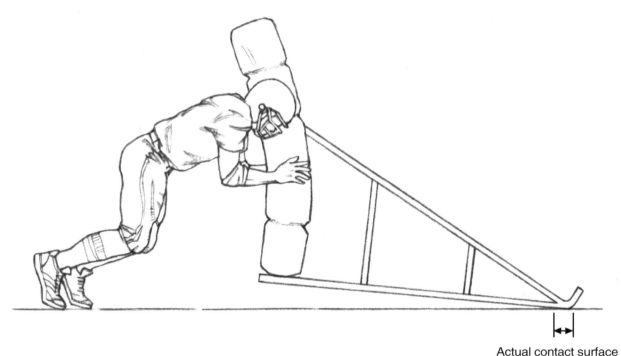

Actual contact surface

Fig. 3.8. Lifting a football blocking sled reduces the actual contact surface.

a contacting or supporting surface. Rolling friction is common, for example, in bowling, billiards, golf, field hockey, cycling, and soccer. The resistive force generated by rolling friction is significantly less (i.e., up to a thousandfold!) than sliding friction. Indeed, use of the wheel is commonplace because of the minimal levels of friction produced as a wheel rolls over a supporting surface. This extremely low-level friction results from the ease with which a rounded surface detaches itself from the surface it is rolling over. Rolling friction varies according to the nature of the surfaces in contact, the pressure pushing the surfaces together, and the diameter of the rolling object.

Rules exist in sport to limit the diameter, mass, and surface of balls and wheels. Coaches and athletes must concentrate on how environmental conditions affect the flight and roll of a ball or the roll of a wheel. In golf, a sport that emphasizes both flight and roll, researchers study the value of using a slightly larger ball (which the rules allow) and varying the number and pattern of the dimples on its surface. Dimples improve the flight characteristics of a golf ball (see chapter 6), but, on the other hand, they increase friction as the ball rolls on a fairway and on greens.

Athletes in sprint cycle races use narrow tubular tires, inflating them to phenomenal pressures that average 120 psi (pounds per square inch). The result is that even with the weight of the cyclist, hardly any tire surface contacts the track, and rolling friction is reduced to a minimum. Even so, the rubber of the tire in contact with the smooth velodrome surface provides excellent traction. It is because of rolling friction that fat-tire mountain bikes feel so sluggish on the road, particularly if their tires are underinflated (see Figure 3.9). On the other hand, wide, knobbly mountain bike tires are designed to produce great stability and traction on rough terrains. High-pressure, narrow tubular tires are virtually useless in these conditions.

Every sport involves friction in some form or another, from the static and sliding friction in gymnastics, ice-skating, and wrestling to the rolling friction in ball games and wheeled sports like cycling, motor racing, and in-line skating. To these types of friction we can add the fluid friction that occurs when objects move through the air and water. Coaches and athletes must know how to make the best use of all the frictional conditions that occur in a sport—what strategies to use when conditions change and what technological innovations to adopt as new materials and designs enter the sport scene. Knowledge of friction's characteristics is requisite to producing optimal performances.

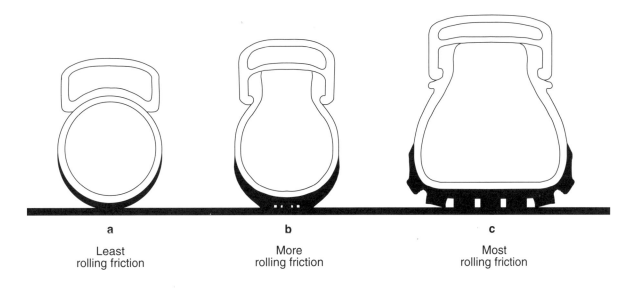

a
Least
rolling friction

b
More
rolling friction

c
Most
rolling friction

Fig. 3.9. Rolling friction increases with the amount of bicycle tire in contact with the road. The least rolling friction occurs with the fully inflated high pressure tubular tire (a). Moderate rolling friction occurs with the fully inflated clincher tire (b), and the most rolling friction occurs with the underinflated mountain bike tire (c).
Reprinted from Chavner and Halstead 1990.

SUMMARY

1. An athlete's acceleration is proportional to the force that the athlete applies (e.g., against the earth) and the time duration the force acts. The product of force multiplied by the time that force acts is called impulse.

2. The acceleration of an athlete or an object is inversely proportional to its mass. For a given impulse, any increase in mass reduces acceleration.

3. All actions cause reactions. Muscular force applied by an athlete against the earth's surface is an action. The earth's push against the athlete is the reaction. Action and reaction are colinear forces, being both equal and opposite.

4. Momentum describes quantity of motion. An increase in mass or velocity increases momentum.

5. Force which is applied to the athlete's body over a large time frame and to a large area helps to avoid injury when athletes come to a stop or when they stop a moving object.

6. Mechanical work is force multiplied by the distance through which force is applied.

7. Power is the rate at which work is done. 550 lb moved 1 ft in 1 sec is 1 horsepower (1 horsepower = 746 watts).

8. There are three types of mechanical energy: kinetic energy, potential energy, and strain energy. Kinetic energy is the energy that an object possesses by virtue of its motion. Potential energy (also called gravitational potential energy) is the energy that an object possesses when at a distance above the earth's surface. Strain energy is the object's capacity to do mechanical work when it recoils after being pulled or pushed out of its normal shape. Strain energy is considered a form of potential energy.

9. The rebound of a ball depends on the elastic recoil of both the ball and the object with which it collides. The velocity of the ball, the angle of impact, and factors like temperature and friction affect the manner in which a ball rebounds.

10. When two objects slide against each other, static friction resists the initiation of motion and sliding friction resists the sliding motion that occurs. Sliding friction is always less than static friction.

11. Four factors affect static and sliding friction: the forces pressing the contacting surfaces together, the actual contact area between the two surfaces, the nature and type of the materials in contact, and the relative motion between the two surfaces.

12. Rolling friction occurs when a round object rolls against a contacting surface. Rolling friction is significantly less than sliding friction. Rolling friction is influenced by the forces pressing contacting surfaces together, the nature and type of the materials in contact, and the diameter of the rolling object.

REVIEW QUESTIONS

1. A soccer ball is kicked at tremendous velocity toward the goal. The goalie standing on the line catches the ball and staggers backward into the goal; the ball loses momentum because it slows down. What gains momentum?

2. Imagine you've been invited to play baseball, but there's no glove for you to use. A batter drives the ball toward you at tremendous velocity. You reach out toward the ball, but don't draw your arm back as you catch it. Why will this be such a painful experience?

3. What happens to the flight path of (a) a ball that is given topspin and (b) a ball that is given backspin? Indicate what part gravity plays in the flight characteristics of the two balls.

4. At the apex of a vault, when for an instant a pole-vaulter is going neither up nor down, what happens to the athlete's kinetic energy? the athlete's potential energy? the strain energy of the pole? the force of gravity?

5. A four-man sled slides slowly at the end of the run. The brakeman applies the brake, and the sled slides a certain distance. With conditions the same on a second run, the sled is sliding twice as fast at the time that the brakeman applies the brake. About how much farther will the sled slide?

6. A gymnast shifts from a two-handed handstand to a one-handed handstand. The pressure that the athlete experiences increases as she shifts from the two hands to one. Why?

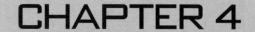

CHAPTER 4

Rocking and Rolling

When you finish reading this chapter, you should be able to explain

■ the factors necessary to initiate and vary angular motion;

■ how athletes apply torque, and how torque varies the rate of spin;

■ how athletes make use of first, second, and third class levers;

■ why rotating objects initially resist rotation and then "want" to continue rotating once they've been set spinning;

■ how the rotary inertia of an object varies;

■ what angular momentum is and how it is determined;

■ how athletes make use of the principle of conservation of angular momentum in such sports as diving, gymnastics, and track and field; and

■ how specific movements, like the body tilt, cat twist, and hula hoop twist, allow athletes to mix somersaults and twists while in flight.

"Rocking and Rolling" is about rotation and it's the largest chapter you'll find in this book. The size of this chapter is an indication not only of the importance of rotation but also of its presence in all sport skills.

The first half of this chapter explains the basic principles that relate to rotation. The second half will be of great interest to those of you wanting to coach gymnasts, divers, and skaters. Here we explain the mechanics of twisting and somersaulting. Even if you don't intend to coach these sports, you will benefit from reading this material because the mechanical principles involved in gymnastics, diving, and skating occur in other sport skills as well.

"Rocking and Rolling" was picked as the title of this chapter because these are words with which we are all familiar. But there's another reason. Rocking and rolling are two of the many terms that coaches use when they refer to angular motion. Coaches also talk of athletes rotating, circling, revolving, spinning, somersaulting, twisting, pirouetting, turning, and swinging. All these terms refer to angular motion.

If you watch closely, you'll see that rotation occurs in all sports, including those that require an athlete to stay as still as possible. In Olympic pistol and rifle shooting for example, athletes try to eliminate all unnecessary movements. They train to slow their heart rates and to pull the trigger between each heartbeat! In this way, the thump of the athlete's heart doesn't jog the barrel of the gun! Even in this slow and patient sport, when the athlete squeezes the trigger the bones of the index finger move in a rotary fashion. It's the same when an archer flexes her arm to pull a bow. As the bowstring is drawn back, forearm and upper arm rotate toward each other. Both shooter and archer hardly move at all, but rotation occurs nevertheless.

Far different from archery and shooting are the sports of gymnastics, diving, ski-aerials, and skating. Dramatic rotary skills performed in flight characterize all these sports. Many of these skills combine somersaults and twists. Divers, ski-aerialists, and gymnasts somersault around their transverse axis (from side to side or from hip to hip) and twist around their longitudinal or long axis (head to feet). Gymnasts also cartwheel and side-somersault around their frontal axis (from front to back) (see Figure 4.1).

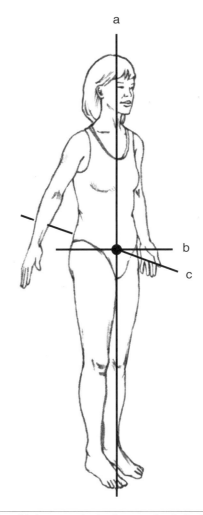

Fig. 4.1. Major axes in the human body include (a) long axis, (b) transverse axis, and (c) frontal axis.

Of all the athletes listed above, gymnasts perform the greatest variety of rotational skills. This is because they compete on many different pieces of apparatus. In contact with stable apparatus (e.g., the floor, beam, vault, bars, pommel horse) and highly unstable apparatus (i.e., the rings), gymnasts perform somersaulting and twisting skills around axes formed by their feet, hands, hips, shoulders, even their knees.

The prize for the greatest number of somersaults and twists performed at any one time belongs not to gymnasts but to ski-aerialists. These daredevil athletes use a "kicker" (i.e., a ramp) that throws them high in the air, and with their flight time extended by a downward sloping "outrun" they combine as many as three somersaults with five twists.

Angular Motion

Angular motion means that an athlete or an object rotates, spins, swings, or twists through an angle of a certain number of degrees. If a gymnast makes one full revolution on the uneven bars, the gymnast has rotated through an angle of 360 degrees. In golf, from windup to follow-through, a golfer can swing a club from 10 to 15 degrees in a putt to more than 360 degrees in a drive. Basketball players who perform "360s" in slam-dunk competitions spin one full revolution around their long axis before slamming the ball through the hoop.

Whether rotation occurs through several revolutions or through an arc of a few degrees, the same mechanical principles apply. It's good to have an understanding of these principles because it helps you teach technique based on sound sport mechanics.

Components of Lever Systems

The use of levers occurs in all sports. To understand how levers work in the human body and to see what part they play in sport, let's look at the components of a lever system (shown in Figure 4.2).

A **lever** is a simple machine that transmits and changes mechanical energy from one place to another. It usually incorporates a fairly rigid object that rocks or rotates around an axis and in so doing produces angular motion. An athlete's muscles, bones, and joints work together as le-

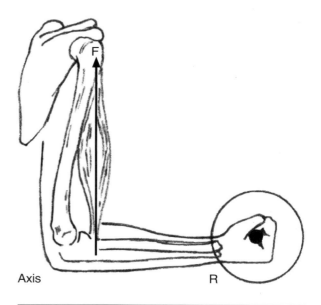

Fig. 4.3. A lever system in the human body. Resistance is the combined weight of the dumbbell and the athlete's forearm.

vers. An axis acts like a hinge on a door, a **fulcrum** on a scale, or an axle of a wheel. In an athlete's body the joints act as axes.

In a lever system, **force** is applied at one location on the lever and a **resistance** applies its own force at another. The action of the applied force helps to make the lever rotate in one direction. The force produced by the resistance tries to make the lever rotate in the opposing direction. Force and resistance battle each other. In an athlete's body, force is primarily produced by muscular contraction. The weight of the athlete's limbs plus the weight of whatever the athlete is trying to move produces resistance. Figure 4.3 shows the position of force and resistance in a dumbbell curl, which is an exercise most athletes use.

The perpendicular distance from where the force is applied, to the axis, is called the **force arm**. Likewise, the perpendicular distance from where the resistance applies its own force, to the axis, is the **resistance arm**. Figure 4.4 shows the force arm and the resistance arm on a lever that has rotated a few degrees. Later in this chapter you'll see that the length of the force arm relative to that of the resistance arm is important in determining what advantage an athlete gains when using a lever.

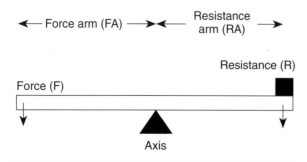

Fig. 4.2. Components of a lever.

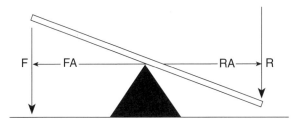

Fig. 4.4. The force arm and the resistance arm on a lever that has rotated a few degrees. The force arm is the perpendicular distance from the force to the axis. The resistance arm is the perpendicular distance from the resistance to the axis.

Torque

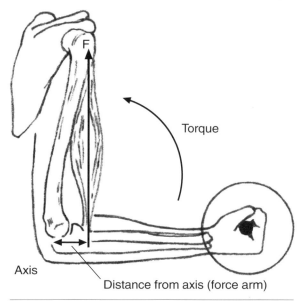

Fig. 4.5. Torque is force multiplied by the perpendicular distance from the axis that force is applied.

Because all levers rock or rotate around an axis, they always produce a turning effect, which we call **torque**. In auto mechanics, a torque wrench is designed to apply a precise turning effect to a bolt. In weight training, a dumbbell curl requires the biceps muscles to pull on the forearm and produce a turning effect, or torque, in an upward direction. How much torque occurs depends on the amount of force produced by the biceps multiplied by the length of the force arm. The force arm is the perpendicular distance from the biceps' attachment on the forearm, to the axis (i.e., the elbow joint) (see Figure 4.5). The dumbbell plus the weight of the athlete's forearm generate their own torque as gravity pulls them down.

To understand how we can increase the turning effect of torque, let's have an athlete become a mechanic and use a wrench to loosen a bolt. When the athlete pulls on the wrench, the athlete applies torque to the bolt. Whether the athlete is successful in overcoming the resistance of the bolt depends on (a) how much force the athlete exerts, (b) how far from the bolt the athlete applies force (i.e., the size of the force arm), and (c) what angle the athlete pulls on the wrench. A 90-degree angle of pull is most efficient.

In Figure 4.6a the athlete applies 10 units of force at 5 units of distance from the bolt (which acts as the axis). The torque produced is 50 units. In Figure 4.6b the athlete applies the same amount of force 10 units of distance from the bolt. In this case the turning effect, or torque, applied to the wrench has been doubled to 100 units because the force arm has been made twice as large. If the athlete wants to produce even more torque, the options available are (a) to apply more force at 90 degrees to the wrench, (b) to increase the size of the force arm, or (c) to combine (a) and (b).

From this example you'll notice that a large force arm is an important requirement if an athlete wants to produce a large amount of torque. Now let's look again at the biceps curl in Figure 4.5. Notice that in producing the turning effect of torque, the biceps has to work with a very small force arm. Later we'll explain how this characteristic (which is common throughout the human body) can be both a disadvantage and an advantage.

The principles followed by the athlete in applying torque to a bolt apply to all lever situations that occur in sport. In essence what happens is a battle between the turning effect of two opposing torques—torque produced by an athlete's muscular forces and torque produced by any type of resistance, such as the weight of the athlete's limbs plus whatever the athlete is holding (e.g., a discus or a barbell). Of course, an opponent can also generate resistance and torque in a sport like wrestling or judo!

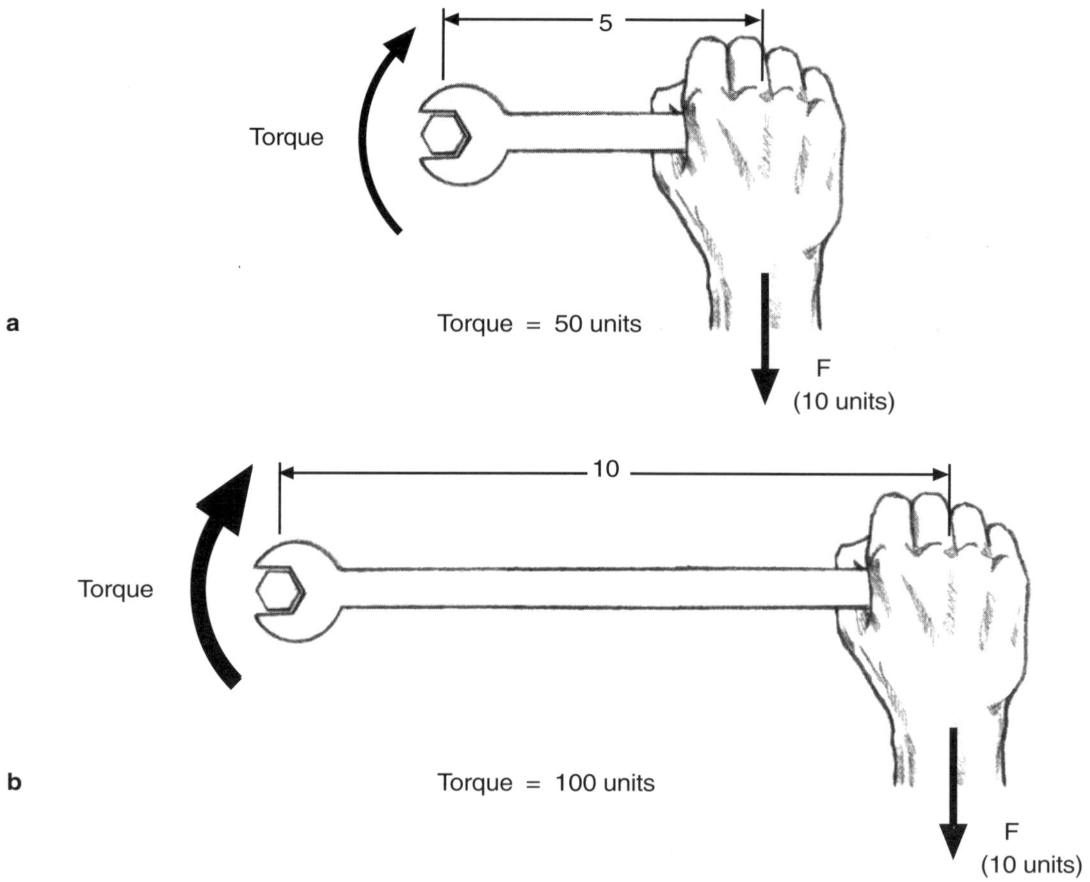

Fig. 4.6. Torque is doubled when force is applied twice the distance from the axis. In (a) force is applied 5 units from the axis, producing a torque of 50 units. In (b) force is applied 10 units from the axis, producing a torque of 100 units.

Sport skills involve many ways to apply the turning effect of torque. To understand these differences let's look at how lever systems can vary.

Types of Levers

Levers are divided into three groups called first, second, and third class. This classification is based on the way the force, resistance, and axis are positioned on the lever relative to each other. In an athlete's body you'll see that third class levers are most common. However, in the performance of sport skills, you'll find that athletes frequently use all three classes of levers.

First Class Levers

In a **first class lever** the axis is situated in between the force and the resistance (see Figure 4.2). The force and resistance arms can be equal in length as they are in the illustration, or they can be unequal. If the force arm is longer than the resistance arm, then the lever favors force output—meaning that the lever arrangement allows the athlete to "get out" more force than the athlete "puts in". If the force arm is shorter than the resistance arm, then the lever favors speed and range of movement at the expense of force. What is lost in force produces a gain in speed and distance, and vice versa. The following examples show how this compromise occurs in sport.

A triceps extension as a first class lever. Figure 4.7 shows a weight training exercise called a triceps extension. In this exercise the contraction of the triceps battles the weight of an athlete's forearm and dumbbell. In this example for ease of explanation, let's forget the weight of the forearm, and consider that the total weight of the resistance is centered in the dumbbell. If the dumb-

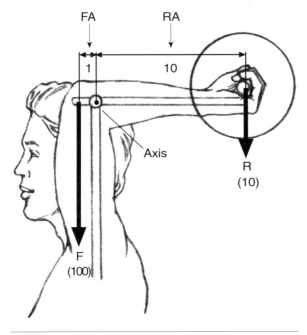

Fig. 4.7. Triceps extension as a first class lever.

bell is 10 lb and the resistance arm 10 units, the triceps working with a force arm of 1 unit must produce a force of 100 lb to hold the dumbbell so it neither rises nor falls. In other words, for equilibrium to exist, force × force arm must equal resistance x resistance arm (i.e., 100 × 1 = 10 × 10). To lift the dumbbell upward the athlete's triceps must produce more than 100 lb of force.

A leg press as a first class lever. First class levers are used frequently in the design of weight training machines. Figure 4.8 shows a simplified illustration of a leg press machine. The athlete applies force on one side of the axis and the weight stack as the resistance applies its own force on the other. On some leg press machines, the athlete will find two sets of foot pedals to push against. One set is purposely positioned lower down on the machine than the other. An athlete who struggles to lift the weight stack using the upper pedals will find it much easier using the lower pedals. Why? Be-

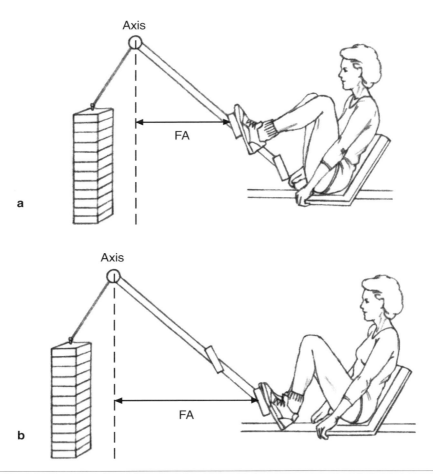

Fig. 4.8. Leg press as a first class lever. When the upper pedals are used, as in (a), the force arm is shortened.

cause on the lower set of pedals the force arm is much longer than on the upper set. This means that the same amount of force applied by the athlete's legs to the lower set of pedals produces greater torque. The turning effect of torque lifts the weight stack. But if something is gained, something has to be lost or given up! The compromise in this situation is that the athlete must push the lower set of foot pedals through a bigger arc of movement than when using the upper set.

Second Class Levers

Second class levers are characterized by having both force and resistance on the same side of the axis, with the force arm always longer than the resistance arm (see Figure 4.9). The applied force acts in one direction and the resistance in the opposing direction. Second class levers favor the output of force at the expense of speed and range of movement. The larger the force arm in relation to the resistance arm the greater the force output. In essence, this means that an athlete who uses a second class lever applies less force over a large distance to shift a heavier resistance a small distance. The following two examples demonstrate these characteristics.

A calf raise as a second class lever. A second class lever can occur when an athlete performs a calf raise with a barbell (see Figure 4.10a). The line of the center of gravity of the athlete and the barbell falls very close to the axis, which is at the athlete's toes or the balls of the feet. An athlete can lift huge poundages with this arrangement because the resistance arm is so small and the force arm so much larger in comparison. However, if the athlete leans forward so the line of the center of gravity of barbell and athlete falls in front of the toes, then the second class lever becomes a first class lever (see Figure 4.10b).

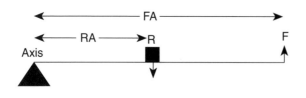

Fig. 4.9. Second class lever.

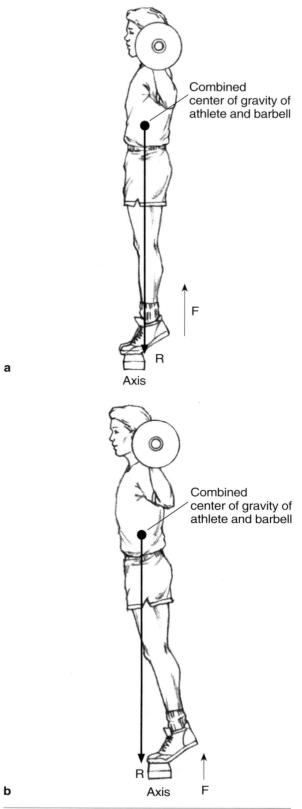

Fig. 4.10. A calf raise can produce a second class lever (a), but leaning forward produces a first class lever (b).

Rowing as a second class lever. In rowing, when the blade of the oar catches the water, the water acts as a temporary shifting axis and the resistance (i.e., the shell plus its occupant) occurs at the oarlocks. The rower provides the force. In this phase of the rowing action, a second class lever is at work (see Figure 4.11). In this example the force arm is the perpendicular distance from where the rower pulls on the oar to where the blade catches the water. The resistance arm is the perpendicular distance from the oarlock to where the blade catches the water. You can see from the illustration that the force arm is much longer than the resistance arm.

Third Class Levers

In a **third class lever** the axis is at one end of the lever and the resistance is at the other end (see Figure 4.12). The applied force acts between the axis and the resistance. Like second class levers, both force and resistance pull or push in opposing directions. Third class levers always move the resistance through a larger range of movement than that moved by the force. On the other hand the force that is applied is always greater than the resistance.

A biceps curl as a third class lever. A biceps curl is a great example of a third class lever because it shows the typical relationship that exists between most of the muscles, bones, and joints in an athlete's body. It also demonstrates how your muscles must exert considerable force even to move a light resistance.

In Figure 4.13 an athlete is holding a dumbbell in a state of equilibrium so that the dumbbell neither rises nor falls. In this situation the upward turning effect (torque) that the athlete's biceps produce equals that caused by gravity pulling downward on the athlete's arm and dumbbell. In this example we have set the ratio of resistance arm to force arm at 10:1. If the resistance is 10 units and the distance to the elbow joint is 10 units, the downward turning effect of the resistance is $10 \times 10 = 100$ units. If the force arm is only 1 unit of distance, the force necessary to hold the forearm and dumbbell horizontal is 100 units, or 10 times that of the resistance.

We must mention one additional characteristic here. With the arm held horizontal, the biceps pulls on the forearm at an angle slightly less than 90 degrees. This arrangement causes some of the force of the biceps to be spent pulling the forearm toward the elbow joint. (Physiologically this helps

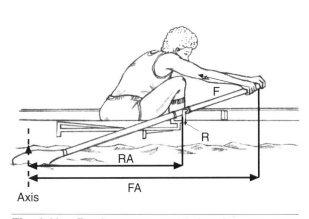

Fig. 4.11.   Rowing as a second class lever.

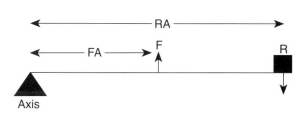

Fig. 4.12.   Third class lever.

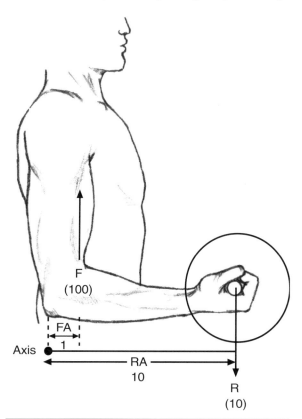

Fig. 4.13.   Biceps curl as a third class lever.

to keep the bones of the elbow joint together.) In Figure 4.14 we have purposely exaggerated the angle of pull of the biceps so that the division of the force produced by the biceps is more apparent. Any angle of pull by the biceps that is not perpendicular to the forearm means that some of the force of the biceps muscle is directed elsewhere (either toward or away from the elbow joint) and so plays no part in producing torque. In Figure 4.14, (a) represents the force produced by the biceps, (b) indicates what part of the force produces torque and lifts the forearm, and (c) shows the force directed toward the elbow joint. What these characteristics tell you is that third class levers coupled with a poor angle of pull put an athlete at a disadvantage in transmitting great muscular force. Whatever force an athlete's muscles produce is greatly reduced by the time it reaches the resistance (which is often an object held in the hand). However, an athlete does gain from this arrangement as you'll see below.

Advantages and Disadvantages of Limb Length

If an athlete contracts the biceps in the curl illustrated in Figure 4.13 so that its attachment on the forearm moves in an arc 1 unit in length, the dumbbell travels around an arc 10 times larger. This increase in range of movement, shown schematically in Figure 4.15, occurs because the resistance arm is 10 times longer than the force arm. Furthermore, if it takes 1 sec for the athlete's

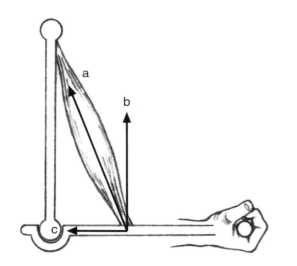

Fig. 4.14. When a muscle (a) pulls at an angle less than or greater than 90°, its force is divided into (b) and (c).

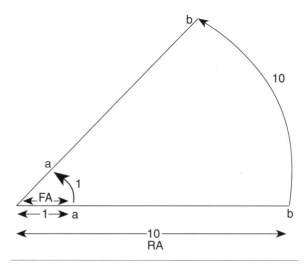

Fig. 4.15. Point (b) on the resistance arm moves 10 times farther and faster than point (a) on the force arm.

Rowers Use Hatchet Blades to Apply More Force

Elite rowers have recently been using oars with huge blades that look like giant meat cleavers. Called "hatchet blades," the new oars are shorter from the oarlock to the blade than standard oars. The mechanical principle behind the new design is that for the same effort, the new blade travels more slowly through the water but applies more force. Moving slower, the blade slips less in the water but propels the shell faster. Do these blades present any problems? Yes. According to many coaches hatchet blades cause stress injuries because the rowers must pull against a stiffer and less mobile resistance.

biceps to complete its arc of 1 unit, the dumbbell moves through an arc 10 times larger in 1 sec also. Thus, the longer the athlete's arm, the faster and farther the dumbbell moves.

These characteristics illustrate the compromise situation that we all experience as a result of the way our bodies are designed. We all suffer because our muscles must exert tremendous force to move a much lighter resistance. Obviously, if we don't have the necessary strength we cannot move even a light resistance. And to make matters worse, the longer our limbs the greater the force required from our muscles. So what do we gain from this arrangement? Think of an athlete with long arms. Long arms mean that an athlete's hand travels at great speed over a huge distance when the arm is swung in an arc. Providing an athlete can generate sufficient force in the muscle, a long limb moves a light resistance (such as a ball or a discus) over an immense range at tremendous speed. This is why discus throwers in the Olympic Games are such huge, long-armed athletes! The more powerful an athlete's muscles and the longer their arms, the better! Short limbs on the other hand, lose less force along their length than do long limbs. You'll see what we mean in the following fantasy competition between former gymnastics great Bart Conner and giant basketball player Shaquille O'Neal!

Let's imagine that Bart Conner and Shaquille O'Neal have similar strength in their pectoral and latissimus muscles. We will ask both athletes to attempt a superdifficult iron cross in the rings.

An iron cross requires an athlete to contract the latissimus and pectoral muscles. These muscles do most of the work in pulling the arms and hands downward on the rings, and simultaneously, as part of their contraction, pulling the body up. This action stops the athlete's body from dropping down out of the cross position.

A basketball player of Shaquille's proportions is immediately at a disadvantage in this skill. Long arms form huge resistance arms. The resistance is Shaquille's body weight which pulls downward. The axis is at his shoulder joint, and his pectorals and latissimus muscles, which provide force, have to work with a very short force arm. (Of course, by being human both Shaquille and Bart suffer from this problem!) The battle becomes force (from Shaquille's muscles contracting) multiplied by a small force arm, versus resistance (his body weight) multiplied by a huge resistance arm (the length of Shaquille's arms).

For Shaquille to hold an iron cross, the turning effect (torque) produced by force × force arm must equal the torque produced by the resistance x resistance arm (see Figure 4.16). Bart Conner with his short arms has a much better chance of success in this skill. Short arms mean short resistance arms, and the torque produced by Bart's lighter body weight working with a short resistance arm is less than that of heavyweight Shaquille with his exceptionally long arms.

Let's consider the issue of body weight for a moment. Shaquille has 300 lb of body weight acting as the resistance. Even though his pectoral and latissimus muscles collectively battle 300 lb of body weight pulling downward, an iron cross would demand strength in these muscles that you'd only find in a "bionic man." The contractile force that Shaquille's muscles would have to produce for an iron cross could even tear them away from where they attach to the bones!

Shaquille's muscles get little help from the short force arm they have to work with, and they fight immense resistance (his body weight) multiplied by a huge resistance arm (the phenomenal length of his arms). These physical characteristics are

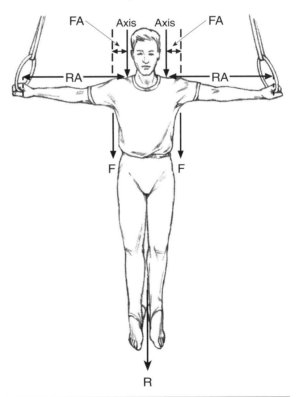

Fig. 4.16. Force arms and resistance arms in the iron cross.

reason enough why Shaquille will stay with basketball and never go near gymnastics!

I'm sure you've noticed that most male gymnasts are around 5' 6" tall and weigh between 120 to 130 lb. Females are even smaller, averaging 5 ft and weighing between 70 and 80 lb. So not only do gymnasts have the advantage of short arms but they also benefit from having minimal body weight. Their resistance arms are short, and their body weight is often less than one half that of basketball players that we see in the National Basketball Association. Success in an iron cross (and other difficult gymnastic skills) is much more likely when you are built like a gymnast. This explains why elite gymnasts are superlight, have short limbs, *and* have to spend much of their time controlling their body weight. A couple of extra pounds can be the difference between success and failure in many gymnastic skills!

Now let's take Shaquille and Bart onto the track to compete against each other in a discus competition. When they throw a discus we find that a taller, heavier, long-limbed athlete has a definite advantage. Figure 4.17 shows the last part of a discus throw. It's easy to see from this illustration that long arms are a great advantage in this event. A spin across the ring by Shaquille with his long arms gives the discus tremendous velocity because it is pulled around a circular pathway made enormous by the length of his arms! Even with a loss of force along the great length of his arms, Shaquille is strong enough to accelerate the light weight of a discus.

Bart loses in the discus event. If both Bart and Shaquille were to spin across the ring at the same rate, a discus in the hand of a long-armed athlete like Shaquille will travel faster. What can Bart do to compensate? He can spin at such a phenomenal rate that he's a blur as he goes across the ring. Obviously this is very difficult to accomplish!

Long arms are a great advantage in an event like the discus and a disadvantage in most gymnastic skills. It depends on what is required by the sport. In some sport skills it is better to be heavy and to have long arms and legs, in other sports they become a disadvantage.

A discus throw as a third class lever. Since we've been putting Bart Conner and Shaquille O'Neal through their paces as discus throwers, it's worth looking at a discus throw as a lever system. Figure 4.17 shows a discus thrower who is just about to release the discus, a good example of a third class lever. The axis of rotation runs from the left foot up through the athlete's body.

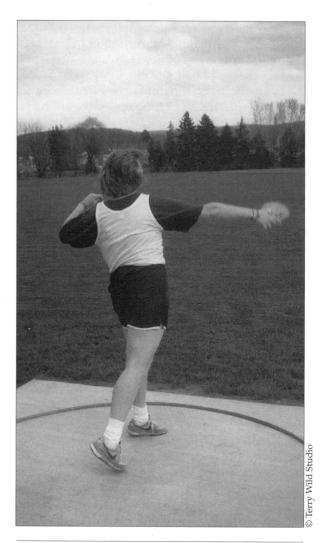

Fig. 4.17.   Discus throw as a third class lever.

Muscular force is produced by the contraction and pull of the thrower's pectoral muscle. The resistance is the discus together with the weight of the thrower's arm.

Initiating Rotation

Recall from our earlier discussion that anytime athletes apply force at a distance from an axis they produce the turning effect of torque. If they increase the distance and/or the force they apply, they make the turning effect greater. The application of torque makes objects and athletes rotate.

In ball games like tennis or volleyball, the server wants to spin the ball on some occasions and avoid spinning it on others. If a great volleyball player like Steve Timmons wishes to serve a floater, he'll make sure that the force he applies to the ball passes directly through the ball's center of gravity, which in flight will be the ball's axis of rotation. When this happens, the ball floats across the net without spinning (see Figure 4.18).

What must happen if Steve wants to spin the volleyball? Then he must apply the force from his hand at some distance from the ball's center of gravity. If Steve increases this distance, it increases spin. Figure 4.19a shows force applied well above the ball's center of gravity. When this happens the ball receives a topspin, and as a result it arcs downward in flight. In golf, a chip shot requires a golfer like Nancy Lopez to apply force well below the ball's center of gravity. The angle of the club face and the stroke technique that Nancy uses does this for her. The ball receives a backspin and lifts in flight (see Figure 4.19b). Depending on the amount of backspin and the surface it lands on, a golf ball can stop dead, or if shot to the far side of the green can roll back toward the pin.

The amount of spin applied to any ball depends on how much force is applied and how far it is applied from the ball's center of gravity. The greater the force and the larger the distance from the center of gravity, the greater the torque and the greater the spin. If you want to apply maximum spin to a football (and you have a big hand), you grip it in the middle where the ball is fattest. Here the force applied by your fingers to the circumference of the ball is farthest away from the ball's center of gravity and its long (i.e., longitudinal) axis. In this way you apply maximum torque, which gives the ball the greatest amount of spin. The drawback with this position is that you put less of your force into throwing the ball for distance. On the other hand, if you want to apply less spin and concentrate on applying maximum force to the ball, you grip it closer to the end (see Figure 4.20, a and b). Most quarterbacks compromise by gripping the ball halfway between these two positions. A bullet passer like John Elway has a tremendously powerful throwing arm and hand. He can apply great torque and directional force to spiral the ball immense distances.

How Athletes Make Themselves Rotate

An athlete who wants to rotate in the air can employ the same method used to apply spin to a volleyball. For example, a gymnast who bounces on a trampoline with his center of gravity directly above the upward thrust of the trampoline bed

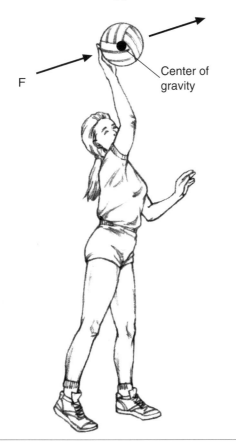

Fig. 4.18. No spin is imparted to a volleyball when force is directed through its center of gravity.
Reprinted from Luttgens et al. 1992.

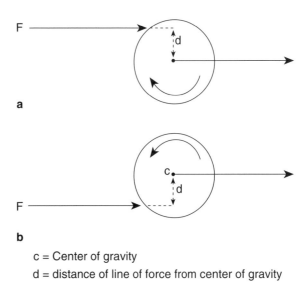

c = Center of gravity
d = distance of line of force from center of gravity

Fig. 4.19. Application of topspin (a) and backspin (b) to a ball.

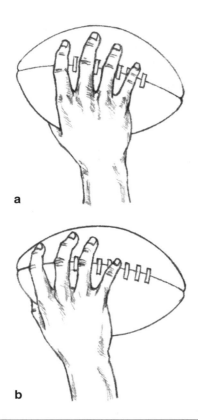

Fig. 4.20. Varying spin and directional force to a football. Grip is in the middle of the ball (a), providing maximal spin and less force for distance. Grip is at the end of the ball (b), providing less spin and maximal force for distance.

rises vertically without rotating. The thrust of the trampoline pushes directly upward through the gymnast's center of gravity. Like the volleyball, the gymnast moves without rotating in the same direction as the thrust of the trampoline (see Figure 4.21a).

If the gymnast positions his center of gravity so that it is no longer directly above the upward thrust of the trampoline bed, there is a tendency to rotate. The more the gymnast shifts his center of gravity out of line with the thrust of the trampoline (i.e., by leaning forward or backward), the greater the turning effect (i.e., torque) applied to his body and the greater the tendency for rotation to occur (see Figure 4.21b).

How Gravity Can Assist With Rotation

Earth's gravitational force (which always acts perpendicularly to the earth's surface) can be used to produce torque and cause rotation. For

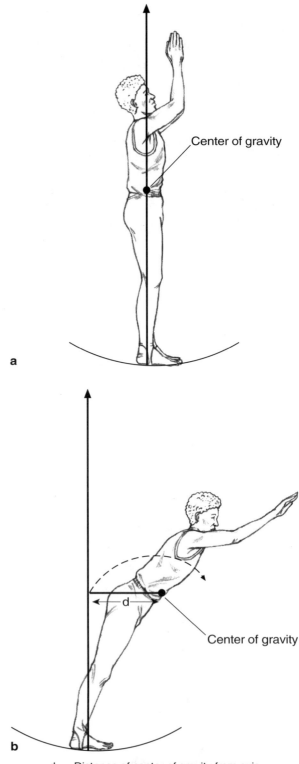

d = Distance of center of gravity from axis

Fig. 4.21. A gymnast rises vertically (a) when the vertical thrust of the trampoline is through the center of gravity. When the thrust from the trampoline does not pass through the gymnast's center of gravity, the torque produced (b) causes the gymnast to rotate.
Adapted from Braecklin 1974.

example, when legendary gymnast Kurt Thomas performs giant circles around a high bar, he is accelerated toward the earth by gravity's pull on the downward portion of the circle. He is then decelerated by gravity on the upward portion.

As Kurt rotates toward the earth, gravity applies torque to his body. The earth's pull is concentrated at his center of gravity and acts perpendicularly downward. The distance (d) of Kurt's center of gravity from the bar, which is the axis around which he spins, is greatest when he fully extends his body in a horizontal position. The greatest turning effect (i.e., torque) applied

by gravity occurs as he passes through this position, because the distance of his center of gravity from the bar is greatest at this point. Conversely, there is no torque produced by gravity when he is directly above or directly below the bar (see Figure 4.22).

In football, a tackle around the ankles can suddenly turn a running back's ankles (or feet) into an axis. The running back rotates around that point. If the running back is sprinting flat out when the tackle occurs, linear motion is dramatically changed into rotation. As the player rotates toward the ground, gravity gets into the act and

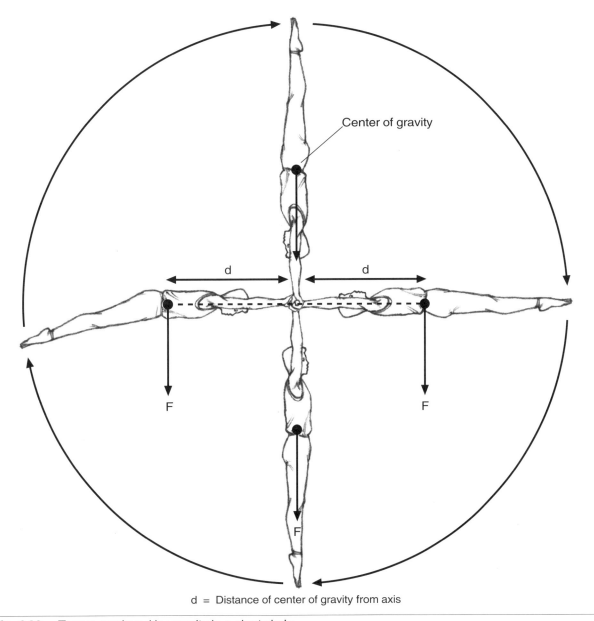

d = Distance of center of gravity from axis

Fig. 4.22. Torque produced by gravity in a giant circle.

assists in accelerating the player downward. The taller the running back, the greater the distance of the player's center of gravity from his feet. So the turning effect is greater too. This is one reason big men fall "heavier" than those not so tall.

Angular Velocity

Angular velocity is a term used to describe the rate of spin of an athlete or an object. These words also describe the rate of swing of a bat or a club. However, there's a difference between the angular velocity and the speed of an object or an athlete as they rotate. To understand the difference let's revisit Kurt Thomas performing giant circles and ask him to rotate around with a perfectly rigid body. (In reality gymnasts have to flex at the hips at specific phases of a giant circle, but for this example, we'll assume that Kurt remains rigid throughout the giant circle).

If you timed Kurt as he went around the bar, your stopwatch might say that he makes one complete revolution in a clockwise direction every second. This information tells you the angle, or the number of degrees (i.e., 360 degrees for each revolution) that Kurt completes in a particular time and in a particular direction.

If you know the number of revolutions, the time frame, and the direction that Kurt is rotating, then you know his angular velocity, or rate of spin. (The word "angular" means angle, degrees, or revolutions, and "velocity" means speed with direction). All parts of Kurt's body make one complete circuit around the bar in a clockwise direction in 1 sec.

Let's now turn our attention to Kurt's body as it rotates. If you watch his hips as they follow their circular pathway, and then watch his feet, you'll come to the following conclusions:

- Kurt's hips travel around a much smaller circle than his feet. His feet, which are farther from the bar, travel around a bigger circle.
- Both Kurt's hips and feet complete their different size circles in the same time frame. So his hips and feet have the same angular velocity.

- If Kurt's feet are twice the distance from the bar as his hips, they travel around a circle that is twice as big and must be moving twice as fast. Their speed is twice that of the hips.

This information tells us that, although all parts of Kurt's body have the same rate of spin (i.e., angular velocity), the farther away from the bar, the faster Kurt's body parts will move. Figure 4.23 shows you that in a giant circle the gymnast's feet (a) move around faster than the gymnast's hips (b), which in turn move faster than the gymnast's shoulders. The gymnast's fingers gripping the bar (c) move slowest of all, yet the fingers have the same angular velocity as all other parts of the gymnast's body. Can you guess by looking carefully at Figure 4.23 which factors influence how fast the gymnast's feet will travel? Their speed depends on how many revs/sec the gymnast rotates (which is the gymnast's angular velocity), and how far the gymnast's feet are from the axis of rotation. (The words "how far" refer to their radius, or distance from the axis of rotation.) The axis of rotation is the high bar itself.

Let's take what we've learned from this high bar example and apply this information to a golf scenario. Imagine that you are getting a lesson from your club pro and the pro tells you, "If you want to drive the ball farther you need to produce more club-head speed . . ." Now you can think to yourself, "OK, for more club-head speed I can increase the angular velocity of my club by swinging it faster through its arc, or I can hold higher up toward the end of the club. This puts the club-head farther from my axis of rotation. By gripping higher on the club I increase the distance (or radius) from my axis of rotation to the club head. Either of these changes will increase the speed of the club-head. Better still, I can do both. That'll give me the most club-head speed" (see Figure 4.24).

You can apply the reasoning that you used during your golf lesson to any sport in which you use bats, racquets, and clubs. If a ball is to be hit as hard as possible, the batter should hold higher up toward the end of the grip to increase the radius and swing as fast as possible. Swinging the bat through its arc as fast as possible means maximizing its angular velocity. Maximum angular velocity combined with the biggest radius possible gives the greatest speed to the striking portion of a club, bat, or racquet.

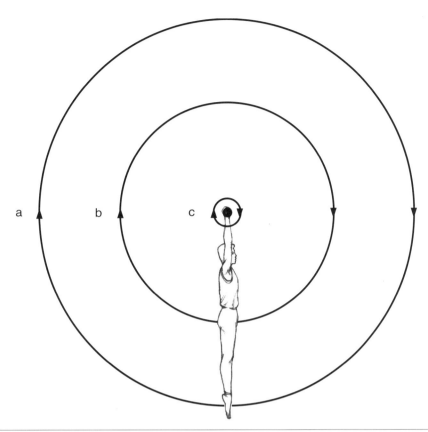

Fig. 4.23. In a giant circle a gymnast's feet (a) travel faster than the hips (b), and the hips travel faster than the hands (c).

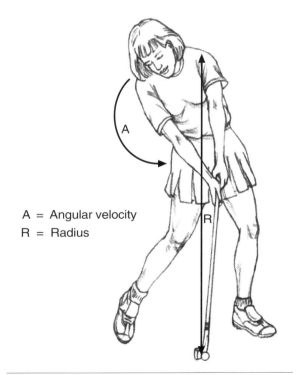

A = Angular velocity
R = Radius

Fig. 4.24. In a golf swing, angular velocity (A) times the radius (R) determine the speed of the club head.

Inertia, Centripetal Force, and Centrifugal Force

Whenever there is rotation, there is always an interplay between inertia, centripetal force, and centrifugal force. All three are present in the spin of a Steve Timmons spike serve, a spiral pass by Steve Young, even a gentle putting stroke by golfing great Greg Norman.

Rotation is a battle between inertia and centripetal force. The inertia of an object when it is moving is expressed in its desire to travel in a straight line. Changing straight-line motion into curved or circular motion requires a centripetal force. This force must pull (or push) the object toward the axis of rotation to make it follow a curved or circular pathway. When an athlete swings a baseball bat, the athlete must apply an inward centripetal force to make sure that the bat follows the arc of the swing. The inward pull of **centripetal force** on the bat produces an outward pull of **centrifugal force** by which the bat pulls on the athlete. All three—

inertia, centripetal force, and centrifugal force—are present when you produce rotation. You cannot have one without the others!

Inertia, Centripetal Force, and Centrifugal Force in the Hammer Throw

To understand how inertia, centripetal force, and centrifugal force are interrelated, let's have the world record holder, Yuri Sedykh of Russia, throw the hammer. Like anything else that has mass, a hammer has no wish to move to begin with, and secondly, no desire to follow a circular path. The inertia of the hammer makes it resist movement. A competitive hammer weighs 16 lb, so it has plenty of mass and consequently a lot of inertia. If Yuri Sedykh applies sufficient muscular force to get the hammer moving around, its inertia will be expressed by its desire to travel in a straight line, not in a circle.

As Yuri spins around in the throwing ring, the ball of the hammer reluctantly follows a big circle at the end of its wire. Most of the mass of a 16 lb competitive hammer is in the ball. There is very little mass in the wire and the handle (see Figure 4.25). To keep the hammer on its circular path, Yuri must continually fight the hammer's desire to get away and travel in a straight line. To do this Yuri constantly pulls inward applying a centripetal force to change the hammer's path from straight to circular. This pull travels from his body, down his arms, along the wire, and out to the hammer ball.

The amount of centripetal force that a hammer thrower must produce depends on what occurs. For example, if an athlete doubles his angular velocity by spinning around twice as fast, he must increase his inward pull on the hammer *fourfold*. Why? Because the hammer goes around twice as fast *and also* pulls on the athlete at every instant on its circular path with twice the force! In other words, an increase in the athlete's rate of spin squares the demand for centripetal force.

What happens if there is no change in the thrower's angular velocity (i.e., rate of spin) but he instead spins around with a hammer twice as heavy? In this case, the athlete must increase his centripetal force *twofold* because the extra mass of the hammer pulls on him at every instant with twice the force. A junior athlete who moves from the 12 lb hammer to the senior 16 lb hammer, or who attempts to spin faster with a hammer of *any* poundage, must be prepared to increase centripetal force by flexing his legs and leaning backward. The weight of his body pushing at an angle against the earth now produces the necessary centripetal force. Failure to carry out this action can throw the athlete off balance and hurl him to the ground!

Why do these changes occur? Because whenever a thrower increases his angular velocity or increases the mass of the hammer, the implement increases its pull on the athlete. During three or four rotations used to throw a hammer, the athlete spins faster and faster. The athlete increases his inward pull on the hammer to hold it to a circular pathway and not let inertia drag it

Technology Gets Involved With the Hammer Throw

The hammer thrown in track and field weighs 16 lb and measures 4 ft from the handle to the farthest point on the surface of the ball. Until the rules were changed, technicians realized that if they used extremely dense tungsten they could put almost all the hammer's 16 lb in the distal portion of the ball. This shifted the hammer's center of gravity farther away from the thrower than a hammer made of less dense material. It also made the ball about the size of a baseball. The handle was then made of superlight titanium so there was virtually no weight in close to the thrower. This "super hammer" was then thrown by an athlete with extremely long arms. Unfortunately there was an unexpected problem! Hammers with 16 lb concentrated in a sphere as small as a baseball buried themselves so deep in the turf that athletes and officials had a hard time pulling them out! Rules now outlaw hammers of this type.

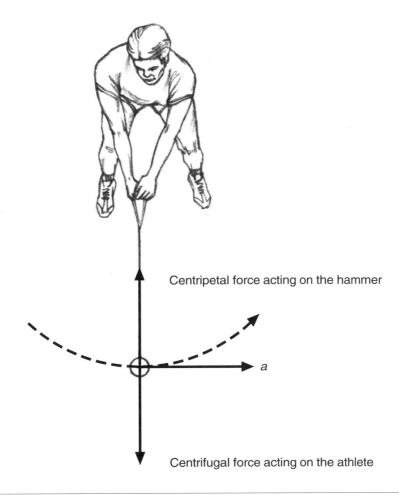

Centripetal force acting on the hammer

a

Centrifugal force acting on the athlete

Fig. 4.25. Centripetal and centrifugal force in the hammer throw. The hammer wants to travel in the direction of arrow *a*.

away on a straight-line path. If the athlete increases his inward pull, the hammer increases its pull on him as well. Spinning around with tremendous angular velocity, the athlete must also lean backward to produce sufficient centripetal force. The right amount of lean balances his pull on the hammer with the hammer's pull on him (see Figure 4.26).

Centrifugal Force

We learned in chapters 2 and 3 that every action causes an equal and opposite reaction. This law doesn't apply only to objects moving in a straight line. It also applies when anything rotates. If an athlete changes the inertial tendency of a hammer to move in a straight line into one that is circular, he must apply a centripetal force by pulling inward on the hammer so that it follows its circular pathway. When he pulls inward there is

an equal and opposite force from the hammer that pulls on him. This is called a centrifugal force which simply means "a force pulling out from the center" (see Figure 4.25). In reality, the athlete has altered the straight-line characteristic of inertia by applying a centripetal force so that the hammer goes around in a circle. When the athlete applies a centripetal force, a centrifugal force occurs also.

The instant the thrower releases the hammer it no longer goes in a circle. If it were not for gravity and air resistance, it would fly away on a straight line path following the trajectory given to it at release. When the thrower releases the hammer, centripetal force immediately disappears and so does centrifugal force. The distance the hammer travels through the air depends on the velocity and trajectory of the hammer ball at the instant of release—not on centripetal and centrifugal force.

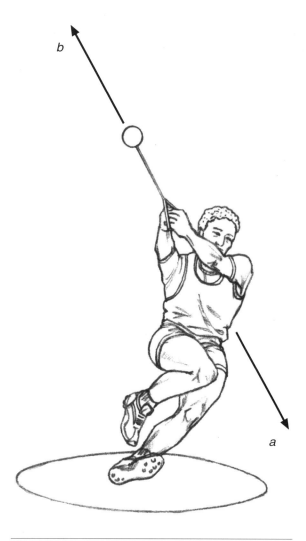

Fig. 4.26.   As the hammer travels faster, the thrower increases centripetal force by leaning away (arrow *a*) from the pull of the hammer (arrow *b*).

Keep in mind that the battle between inertia and centripetal force occurs in all sport skills in which there's rotation and not just in hammer throwing. For example, when a world champion speed skater like Bonnie Blair speeds around the oval and leans into each curve, she obeys the same principles as the hammer thrower when he leans backward. By leaning, she pushes at an angle on the earth. The earth pushes back (equal and opposite) and provides the inward push of a centripetal force. The faster she travels around the curve, and the tighter the curve, the more she must lean and push outward against the earth to get the earth to push her inward!

The fact that Bonnie has to push outward to get around the curve indicates that some of her force is used pushing outward while the remainder is used to propel her forward along the ice. Once she's out of the curve, then all her force can be used in driving her toward the finishing line. The same situation faced sprinter Florence Griffith Joyner when she flashed around the 200 m curve to set her unbelievable world record of 21.34 sec. Compared with running on a straight-away where all the sprinter's effort can be spent driving toward the tape, running a curve makes the athlete spend some precious energy thrusting outward to get around the curve. Proof of this division of effort shows up in comparing the records for 220 yd on the straightaway and 200 m on a curve. (Keep in mind that 220 yd is 1.28 yd *longer* than 200 m!) Peter Brancazio (1984) tells us that in 1966 Tommie Smith ran the 220 yd on a straightaway in 19.5 sec. Yet, until 1996, Pietro Mennea of Italy held the world record for the 200 m around a curve at 19.72 secs. At the 1996 Atlanta Games, the USA's incredible Michael Johnson ran 19.32 secs. Can you imagine what times he'd run on a straightaway?!

Is there any way in which a sprinter can get help in negotiating the curve? Yes, bank the curves. A banked track pushes the athlete inward the same way that the spin cycle of a washing machine holds clothes to a circular pathway, yet allows the water in the clothes to fly outward! On tight indoor tracks, high banking allows the athletes to run flat out without fearing that their inertia will cause them to fly off and in among the spectators! Outdoor tracks are not normally banked, so the tight inside lanes can be difficult to negotiate. This is particularly the case for heavier sprinters who have more inertia and must push outward more vigorously to get their extra body mass around the curve.

Rotary Inertia

Rotary inertia can be thought of as "rotary resistance" and "rotary persistence." It's a term applied to the tendency of all objects or all athletes initially to resist rotation and to want to continue rotating once they have had the turning effect of a torque applied against them. This mechanical principle occurs in every situation in which athletes rotate, spin, or twist, and in every situation in which bats, clubs, and other implements are swung. In short, rotary inertia exists in all sporting situations where angular (i.e., rotary) motion

Gentle Curves Help Set World Records

Most of the world records set in 1988 at the speed skating oval in Calgary were broken during the 1994 Winter Olympics at the oval in Lillehammer, Norway. The total distance around the Hamar and Calgary ovals is the same, but, as you can see from the following measurements, the curves at Hamar are not as tight as at Calgary.

Calgary   Curve radius to inside edge of outside lane = 95 ft
Curve radius to inside edge of inside lane = 83 ft

Hamar   Curve radius to inside edge of outside lane = 97 ft
Curve radius to inside edge of inside lane = 84 ft

Were the athletes helped by the differences in size of the curves at either end of the speed-skating ovals? Yes! On the larger radius curves at Hamar, less of the skater's energy was spent fighting inertia's desire to have the athlete "fly outward" and slam into the crash pads around the outside edge of the curve. As a result, speed skaters were able to take the turn faster and enter the straightaway faster as well.

occurs. Rotary inertia is the rotary equivalent of linear inertia. Here's an example of the relationship of the two. A massive lineman has great linear inertia. If this lineman got on a merry-go-round (like those you find in your local playground), it would require a lot of effort (i.e., force) from a friend to get the merry-go-round spinning. But once underway, the merry-go-round (with the added mass of the lineman) wants to continue spinning! If the lineman's teammates got on as well, they would increase the merry-go-round's rotary inertia even further. Together they act like a giant flywheel. They'd need a lot of force to get themselves spinning, but once underway all their mass (with that of the merry-go-round) would want to keep spinning! Do you see how this illustrates rotary resistance before rotation occurs and rotary persistence once rotation has been initiated?

There are two important factors that determine how much inertia a rotating object will have. These factors are the following:

1. **The mass of the object.** The more mass an object has the more resistance it puts up against being rotated. In addition, the more mass the greater the persistence the object has in wanting to continue rotating once rotation is established. A heavy (i.e., more massive) baseball bat is more difficult to swing than a light one. It resists being accelerated through the swing more than the lighter bat. Once a batter has applied sufficient turning effect, or torque, to get a bat moving, a heavy bat wants to continue the swing more than a lighter one. The heavier the bat, the stronger an athlete must be to get it moving and to control and stop it once this motion has been initiated.

2. **The radial distribution of mass.** The term **radial distribution of mass** refers to how the mass of an object is distributed, or positioned, relative to the axis around which it's spinning. Two extremes in the distribution of mass are whether the object's mass is far from the axis of rotation, or whether it is close to the axis of rotation.

Here's an example of how radial distribution of mass occurs in sport situations. Imagine that you were given two golf clubs. We'll call them club A and club B. The two clubs are alike in length and shape, and on a scale they weigh exactly the same. Club A is like any other golf club that you would buy in a sports store. But as soon as you pick up club B you know that it differs tremendously from club A. Except for a couple ounces of weight in the shaft, all of its weight (i.e., mass) has been concentrated in the club head. Club B will have more rotary inertia than club A because all of its mass is way out in the club head! Compared with club A, you'll find that a swing with club B will be more difficult to initiate. It will also be more difficult to control during the swing and more difficult to stop once the swing is underway.

Now let's take club B, with all of its weight (i.e., mass) in the head, and start repositioning its mass by shifting it up the shaft of the club toward the grip. Suppose this is done in a series of steps by sawing off most of the club head and binding it with tape partway up the shaft. As the club's mass is progressively moved up toward the grip, its rotary resistance (or rotary inertia) is gradually reduced so it becomes easier to swing and easier to control. When all of its mass is in the grip, the club will feel like a fencing foil, which has most of its weight in the handle. You'll feel that you can maneuver it easily, but you'll also know that a club designed in this fashion will never hit a golf ball very far!

How Differences in Distribution of Mass Vary Rotary Inertia

We have just seen that the rotary inertia of any object, whether it is a golf club or an athlete, depends on how much mass it has (the more mass, the more rotary inertia) and how its mass is positioned relative to its axis of rotation (the farther the mass is from the axis of rotation, the greater the rotary inertia). How does this relationship work?

For every distance unit that mass is moved in or out from the axis, the effect on rotary inertia is squared. Here's how this phenomenon works. Imagine that we have a ball with every particle of its mass concentrated at its center. (Of course no ball ever has *all* of its mass at its center, but for this example let's consider that one exists!) In Figure 4.27a the ball is on a string and rotating around an axis at 1 rev per sec. The distance of the ball from the axis is 2 units. In Figure 4.27b, this distance is

halved so it is reduced to 1 unit. This reduction in radius causes the rotary inertia of the ball to be reduced fourfold. Because of this, the ball finds it easier to rotate and it speeds up (i.e., increases its angular velocity) proportionally from 1 rev to 4 revs/sec. In Figure 4.27c, the distance of the ball from the axis has been doubled from 2 units to 4. The rotary inertia of the ball is now increased fourfold. The ball finds it more difficult to rotate and slows to 1/4 rev/sec.

In sport there's no situation in which *every* little bit of an object or an athlete is shifted toward or away from its axis. You cannot move every particle of a baseball bat to one end, because there would be nothing left to make up the remaining part of the bat! Nor can you shift every particle of a bat halfway along its length because that leaves nothing at the ends. It's the same with athletes.

But there is a big difference between athletes and inanimate objects like baseball bats! Athletes can change their shape at will. They can tuck their bodies up tight, or they can extend them. By carrying out these maneuvers, they pull their masses in close to their axes of rotation, or they extend their bodies and push them out as far away from their axes of rotation as possible. Let's see how this occurs in diving.

Manipulating Rotary Inertia in Diving

When great divers like Greg Louganis somersault in the air and move from an extended body position to a tuck, they flex their torsos, legs, and arms, and tuck in their heads. Some parts of their body (i.e., their arms and legs) shift in toward their transverse axis (hip to hip) a large distance. Other parts like their head move in a short distance. Nevertheless, there is still a dramatic difference in rotary inertia between an extended and tucked body position. A diver's legs and the arms are relatively

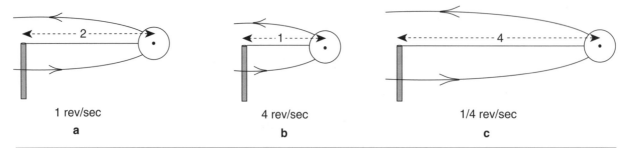

Fig. 4.27.   Reducing the radius from 2 units (a) to 1 unit (b) reduces rotary inertia fourfold. Doubling the radius from 2 units (a) to 4 units (c) increases rotary inertia fourfold. (Air resistance and gravity have been discounted.)

heavy and constitute a lot of body mass. They move in toward the diver's axis a large distance so they have a big effect in reducing the resistance of the diver's body against rotation.

When divers are in flight and in an extended body position, you'll see that they rotate slowly. If they pull their bodies into a tight tuck, they rotate much faster. The more body mass they pull toward their axis of rotation (which passes through their center of gravity) the faster they spin. This means that a lean body coupled with great flexibility plays an important role in determining how much faster divers spin when they pull into a tuck. Huge, muscular (or obese) athletes have a tough time pulling themselves in as tight as lean athletes. Their excess body mass gets in the way! That's one reason today's great Chinese divers look positively skinny! With little to no excess body mass, they pull themselves into the tightest tuck possible. The technique they use for multiple somersaults is similar to that used by trapeze artists. Trapeze artists perform quadruple somersaults by gripping their shins and pulling the knees up as high as possible toward their shoulders. The more compressed and compact they are, the faster they spin (see Figures 4.28, a and b).

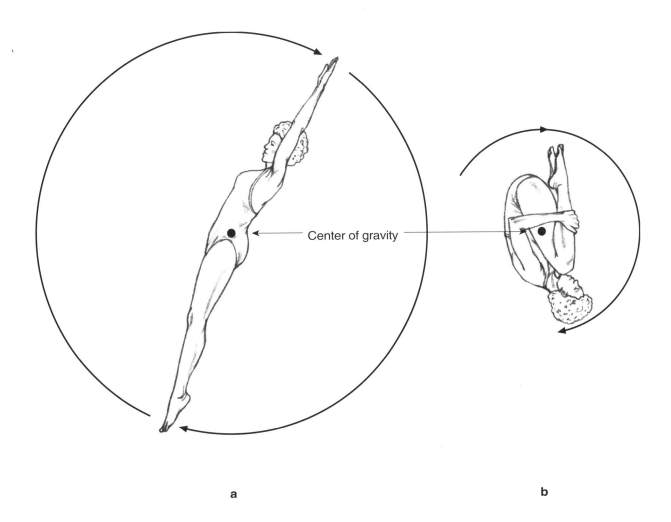

Center of gravity

a

b

Fig. 4.28. Angular velocity increases as the diver (a) pulls her body in close (b) to her axis of rotation (which in flight passes through her center of gravity).

Rotary Inertia in Sprinting

Athletes vary their rotary inertia in many events, not just in sports like diving. For example, in sprinting 100 m, a sprinter extends the legs to the rear of the body and flexes them when they come forward for the next stride. Likewise, when the legs are driven forward, the thigh is elevated and the leg flexed at the knee. Flexing at the knee brings the mass of the sprinter's leg closer to the hip joint (which is the axis around which the leg rotates). This reduces the leg's rotary inertia. If the rotary inertia of the leg is reduced, it makes the task of moving the leg forward much easier for the muscles involved (see Figure 4.29).

Angular Momentum

Angular momentum refers to mass that is rotating, spinning, or turning. More precisely, the two words describe the quantity of motion that a rotating athlete or an object possesses. In sport it's often important for athletes to generate as much angular momentum as possible, whether it's to their own bodies, to an opponent, or to a bat or a club. On other occasions, athletes must reduce

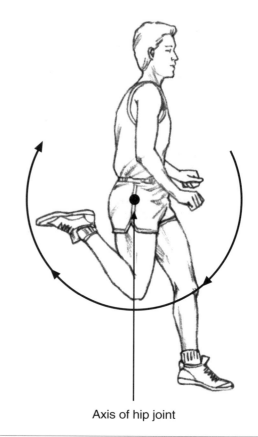

Axis of hip joint

Fig. 4.29. Rotary inertia of the sprinter's leg is reduced when it is flexed.

Olympic Pole Vault Differs From Dutch Canal Vaulting

One of the rules in pole vault says that a vaulter cannot shift the upper handhold. Why? Because in the old days, vaulters were monkey-climbing the pole! If you visit Holland, you'll see a competition in which climbing the pole still occurs. The Dutch pole-vault *for distance* across water-filled canals. Climbing the pole gives them more distance and a dry landing on the other side of the canal. If they climb the pole too soon, they can stall and drop in the water, or even fall back toward the takeoff. Spectators love the drama and the inevitable dunkings! When they climb the pole, the vaulter's rotation slows. Why? Because as they raise themselves upward, vaulters move their mass away from the pole's axis and they increase their rotary inertia. A musician's metronome does the same thing. Raise the weight and the metronome clicks at a slower tempo. Keep raising the weight and the metronome will stop altogether.

angular momentum to minimal values. To help you understand how angular momentum is used in sport, let's review linear momentum, and then we'll look at angular momentum.

In chapter 3 we used a football lineman charging straight ahead as an example of linear momentum. The more massive the lineman and the faster he moves, the more momentum he produces. We can apply the same concept to objects that rotate, or to rotating objects (like bats being swung) that meet objects like baseballs being pitched.

In baseball, a pitch travels in a predominately linear manner to meet a bat moving in an arc. The ball has linear momentum, and if it spins, it has some angular momentum too. The bat being swung has angular momentum. Even if a pitcher hurls a fastball at 100 mph, the ball will still not have much momentum because it doesn't weigh much and so doesn't have much mass. The bat swinging around its arc at a slower speed is much more massive than the ball and so has more momentum. At impact, the ball changes direction and is driven backward.

Suppose a pitcher could fire the ball over the plate at 1,000 mph! In this situation, even though the mass of the ball has not changed, its velocity has increased tremendously, and as a result its momentum has increased too. In this imaginary situation, the ball could have more momentum at impact than the bat. The bat will be driven back or, if it's made of wood rather than aluminum, it could snap off at the handle.

What can a coach do to compete against a pitch traveling at 1,000 mph? Go searching again for a bionic man who's a cross between Reggie Jackson and Arnold Schwarzenegger and who can swing a massive bat at phenomenal speed! Design the bat to have a large amount of its mass (i.e., weight) concentrated at the sweet spot where it contacts the ball. If our bionic man can react fast enough for a 1,000 mph pitch, the bat will win instead of the ball. In all likelihood the ball will disappear out of the park and land in the next city!

This fantasy scenario gives us some idea of the components that make up angular momentum. These components are as follows:

- Mass (i.e., how massive the object is)
- How the mass is positioned relative to the axis the object is spinning around
- The rate of rotation, or swing (i.e., its angular velocity)

In reality, when clubs and bats are swung, there's always a trade-off between the mass of the bat, its length and mass (weight) distribution, and the rate at which the bat is swung. In baseball, no slugger on record has used a bat 42 in long, which is the limit the rules will allow. Batters tend to use bats weighing between 32 and 34 oz though there are no legal restrictions on using a heavier one. The reason? A huge, long, heavy bat with most of its mass in the barrel end demands tremendous power from the batter and inevitably takes longer to accelerate than a light bat. The speed of a pitch gives a batter only a fraction of a second to react. So batters opt for a lighter bat that they can swing quickly. Perhaps they also know that the angular velocity of the bat (i.e., its rate of swing) is more important than how massive the bat is in determining how far a baseball will travel!

The importance of generating as much angular momentum as possible occurs in sports in which athletes rotate, just as much as in sports in which bats and clubs are swung. In diving, particularly in those dives that require numerous twists and somersaults, it is important that the diver generate both linear and angular momentum at takeoff. The diver uses linear momentum to get high above the board and sufficiently far enough away from the board to be safe. At the same time the diver must initiate rotation at takeoff and make sure that her body is extended and spread out. By extending and spinning, the diver has produced angular momentum. The diver can use this angular momentum to help perform all the somersaults and twists that occur later in the dive.

Increasing Angular Momentum

The batting example we looked at earlier indicates that it's possible to increase angular momentum in three ways:

1. Increase the mass of whatever is rotated. Athletes can choose a heavier bat to swing. If athletes are rotating, they must suddenly (and magically!) gain weight to increase angular momentum. Obviously, this is not possible!
2. Shift as much mass as far from the axis of rotation as possible. If athletes are rotating, they must extend their bodies. If they are swinging a bat, it must be long and with most of its mass at the barrel end.

3. Increase the angular velocity of whatever is rotated. Athletes can increase their rate of spin. Batters can swing a bat faster and so give it more angular velocity.

Keep in mind that you always have to find a balance between mass, distribution of mass, and angular velocity. In striking and hitting skills, a huge increase in mass placed a long way from the axis of rotation is like putting a superheavy boot on the kicking foot of a field goal kicker. If the athlete doesn't have the strength to swing his leg, the extra mass is worthless. The right amount of mass combined with a long leg and tremendous angular velocity is what's required.

Using Angular Momentum at Takeoff

The rules of high jump demand that athletes jump from one foot. A two-footed takeoff is not allowed. If the world's first 8 ft leaper, Javier Sotomayor of Cuba, pushed down on the earth with one leg and did nothing else, he'd not go very high! What Javier adds to the thrust of his jumping leg is a strong upward swing by the arms and his free leg. By performing these actions, Javier generates angular momentum that is then transferred to his body as a whole. The upward swing of the arms and free leg adds to the thrust of the leg that is pushing down on the earth. More push down at the earth means that the earth in reaction pushes the athlete more too! The result is that he gets higher into the air (see Figure 4.30).

When world all-around gymnastic champion Vitaly Shcherbo performs a back somersault, he uses a similar technique as Javier Sotomayor. He swings his arms upward to assist in getting up off the ground. For greatest effect, the arms are extended and swung upward with tremendous velocity.

Elite high jumpers and gymnasts always make sure that their takeoff actions occur while in contact with the earth. Skaters do the same. The ice is simply an extension of the earth. Great skaters push against the ice because the ice is part of the earth and the more they push, the more the earth pushes back against them. If they push down, the earth pushes them up! It's this reciprocal response from the earth that gets the skaters up in the air for their triples and quadruples.

If athletes try the same actions while in the air and not in contact with the earth, a totally

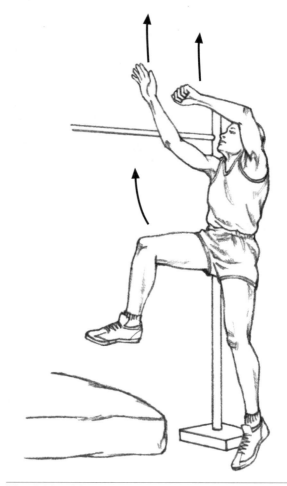

Fig. 4.30. Momentum transfer in a high jump takeoff.

different effect occurs! We discuss this in the following sections.

Conserving Angular Momentum

The word "conserve" means to stay the same, to be conserved, or to be maintained. These words apply to the amount of angular momentum that an athlete possesses during a particular phase of a skill. For example, the angular momentum an athlete generates at takeoff in high jump, long jump, and diving remains the same while the athlete is in flight. Why? Because athletes cannot push against the air to increase or decrease their angular momentum, and during flight the air has a negligible effect in reducing their angular momentum. The only force that's working on the athlete is the earth's gravitational force, which pulls at the athlete's center of gravity. This force doesn't have any effect on the athlete's angular momentum, although gravity increases the athlete's linear momentum as it accelerates the athlete toward the earth. Consequently the athlete's angular momentum doesn't increase or decrease. It stays as is. This means that the angular momentum generated at takeoff is conserved during flight. Let's look at diving again and see how the **conservation of angular momentum** is tied in with a diver's ability to control the rate of spin while in the air.

Controlling the Rate of Spin in Diving

When divers accelerate down from the 10 m tower, it takes less than 2 sec to hit the water. In flights of such short duration the divers' angular momentum is conserved. The amount of angular momentum generated at takeoff stays virtually the same throughout the dive.

In flight divers, just like gymnasts, shift from layout body positions to tight tucks. To get to the latter position a diver uses muscular force to pull the legs and arms inward, to tuck in the chin, and to flex the spine. By carrying out these actions the diver pulls her mass closer to the axis of rotation. When this happens, rotary inertia (i.e., the diver's resistance against rotation) is reduced and the diver spins faster (i.e., the diver's angular velocity increases). But what causes the diver to spin faster? Where does the extra angular velocity come from? The answer is found by examining what happens when one of the items that makes up angular momentum is increased or decreased.

We know that the amount of angular momentum the diver possesses in flight is determined by the diver's rate of spin, the diver's mass, and finally, the distribution of the diver's mass. In other words, how much spin, how much mass, and how extended or balled-up the diver is. All three of these factors combine to make up the diver's angular momentum.

If a diver is in a situation (e.g., in flight) in which the diver's total angular momentum *stays at a set amount* and one factor creating angular momentum is reduced (e.g., the diver tucks and pulls her body mass inward), then another component of angular momentum must increase to keep the total angular momentum unchanged. Since a diver cannot possibly change her mass (i.e., gain or lose weight) while in flight, it means that when she tucks and pulls herself in toward her axis of rotation, the result is that her angular

velocity increases. Pull your body inward and you spin faster. Spread your body out and you spin slower.

Controlling the Rate of Spin in Skating

Another example of athletes reducing rotary inertia by pulling themselves in tight to increase the rate of rotation occurs when an ice-skater performs a multiple twisting skill in the air like a Lutz or an Axel. In these skills a skater completes several rotations (i.e., twists) around the long axis (head to feet) during flight. During the short time that the skater is in flight the athlete's angular momentum is conserved.

A skater drives up into an Axel with one leg forward and the other back. The arms are extended sideways. As a result, the skater's body mass is spread out relative to the long axis of the body. (This is like the diver being extended at takeoff from the board.) In a spread out position the skater's rotary inertia (resistance) is considerable, and so the skater's angular velocity (i.e., rate of spin) around the long axis is minimal. But in flight the skater pulls the arms and legs inward, which greatly reduces resistance against rotation. The skater now twists with tremendous angular velocity. When the arms and legs are spread out again the skater's rotary inertia is again increased and the rate of spin reduced.

The main features of the principles discussed above apply even when a skater performs high speed spins while remaining in contact with the ice. The rate of spin is increased as the skater pulls the limbs inward. The difference between this situation and a skill performed in the air is that a skater's blades pressing and turning on the ice generate more resistance than the air does when the skater is in flight. So a skater loses some angular momentum because the skates experience friction with the ice.

Making Use of Angular Momentum During Flight

When a diver like Greg Louganis is in flight, there is no large mass like the earth for him to push against. Any muscular action that he performs while in the air causes an equal and opposite reaction to occur elsewhere in his body. All divers, gymnasts, and other high-flying athletes experience this characteristic. For example, imagine Greg stepping off the tower and dropping toward the water in an upright position. In this position Greg is not rotating. As he drops, imagine Greg's coach shouting for Greg to raise his legs 90 degrees from perpendicular (i.e., pointing directly downward) to horizontal. The muscles that rotate Greg's legs forward and upward around the hip joint pull equally at both origin and insertion (i.e., at either end of the muscle), and so simultaneously pull down on his trunk. The result is that during the time frame that Greg's legs rotate upward, his trunk must rotate downward. Do Greg's legs and trunk rotate toward each other in equal size arcs? No, because they do not have the same rotary inertia. The rotary inertia of his trunk and upper body is approximately three times that of his legs. So Greg's trunk and upper body resist rotation three times more than his legs. When Greg's legs move upward 90 degrees to a horizontal position, his trunk and upper body, which have three times more rotary resistance than the legs, move downward in an arc a third of the size, or approximately 30 degrees (see Figure 4.31).

The difference between the movement of Greg's legs compared with that of his trunk and upper body may not seem like an equal and opposite reaction, yet it is! In our example, the action is the 90-degree arc moved upward by Greg's legs. The reaction is the 30-degree arc moved downward by his trunk and upper body. This reaction is equal because Greg's trunk and upper body have three times the rotary inertia of his legs. It is opposite because the movement of the trunk and upper body is in the opposing direction to that of the legs.

We've seen that rotary inertia depends not only on how much mass but also how it is distributed relative to its axis. In the example above, Greg kept his legs extended throughout their 90-degree movement. If on the other hand, he flexes at the knees and lifts his thighs, then the rotary inertia of his legs is reduced. The reaction of his trunk and upper body is also reduced. Greg's upper body and trunk flexes forward approximately 20 degrees (see Figure 4.32).

Figure 4.33 shows that another reaction will occur in Greg's movements. As you look at the illustration you will notice that as Greg's extended legs rotate counterclockwise, his trunk and upper body rotate clockwise. In the illustration, these body parts move toward the right as

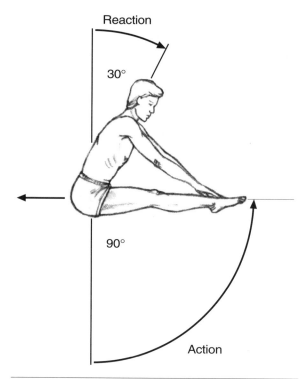

Fig. 4.31. When the diver's extended legs are raised 90° in a counterclockwise direction, the upper body reacts by moving 30° in a clockwise direction.

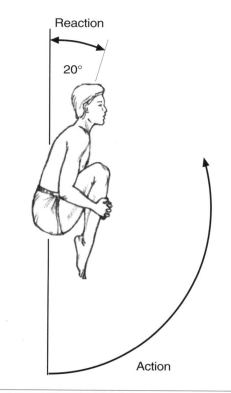

Fig. 4.32. When the diver's flexed legs are raised, they have less rotary inertia than when they are raised in an extended position. The upper body response is less.

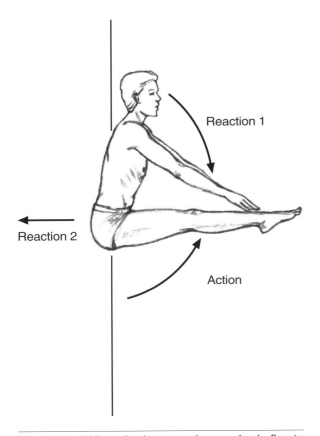

Fig. 4.33. When the lower and upper body flex to the right, the hips react by shifting to the left.

you look at them. In the air, body parts moving to the right are counterbalanced by other body parts moving to the left. In our example Greg's seat and hips react (equal and opposite) by moving toward the left.

This interesting phenomenon of equal and opposite reactions occurring in the air is visible in many sports. A flop jumper always arches to clear the bar. Figure 4.34 shows a flop jumper arching the upper body down toward the pit in a counterclockwise direction. The legs respond (equal and opposite) by moving in a clockwise direction. Although upper body and legs are moving in opposing directions, both are moving down toward the pit. The hips react by moving upward. Correctly timed, a flop jumper uses this action when passing over the bar. The athlete's hips and seat move upward and this helps in clearing the bar.

Another example of this phenomenon occurs when a volleyball player jumps to spike a ball (see Figure 4.35). As the upper body flexes backward in a counterclockwise direction, the lower body reacts by moving in a clockwise direction. As you look at the illustration, you will see that although the upper and lower body are rotating in opposing directions, both move to the left. An equal an opposite reaction must balance this

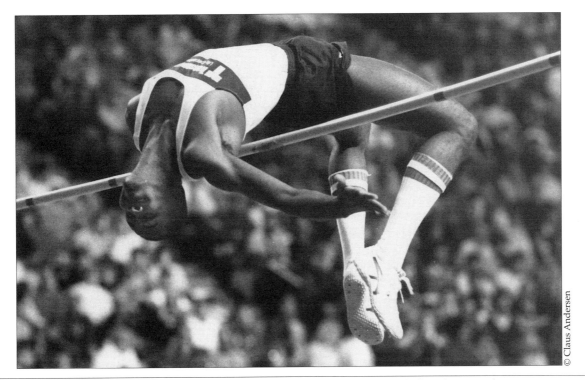

© Claus Andersen

Fig. 4.34. The high jumper's hips lift upward when the upper and lower body flex downward.

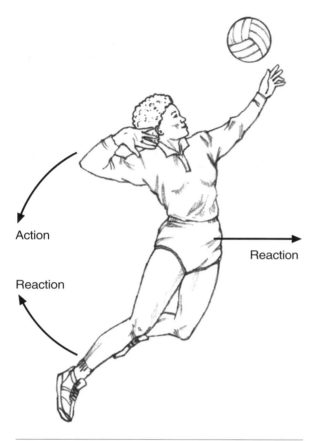

Action

Reaction

Reaction

Fig. 4.35.   Action and reaction in a volleyball spike.

movement. The hips and abdomen shift in the opposing direction. Do you see how this replicates the action of the flop high jumper?

In events like the long jump, high jump, skating, diving, and gymnastics, the athlete is only in the air for a short time. During flights of short duration we know that the athlete's total angular momentum remains constant. If an athlete introduces more angular momentum during flight by suddenly rotating the arms or legs, this additional angular momentum means that another part of the body (or the body as a whole) has to give up some angular momentum to keep the total constant. In other words, if world heptathlon champion Jackie Joyner-Kersee gives herself 10 units of angular momentum at takeoff in one of her jumping events she cannot increase this 10 units to 12 while in flight. If 2 units of angular momentum are introduced by Jackie rotating her arms and legs, then 2 units have to disappear somewhere else in her body to keep the total constant at 10!

Interestingly enough, this principle gives athletes some control over movement in the air. Let's

first look at what occurs in ski jumping, then we'll take a closer look at the long jump where elite jumpers put this principle to good use.

In ski jumping, a jumper who mistakenly gives himself too much forward rotation at takeoff knows that unless something is done about the problem he's likely to land on his face! So the ski jumper desperately rotates his arms *in the same direction* as the unwanted forward rotation. The angular momentum generated by the arms helps to put the brakes on the forward rotation of his body. If performed vigorously enough, the arm action can rotate the skier's body backward into a more favorable position. If the skier rotated the arms backward, his body would rotate farther forward, which in the situation we've described is the last thing he wants to do!

Controlling Forward Rotation in Long Jump

All long jumpers rotate forward at takeoff. Even great jumpers like Carl Lewis, Jackie Joyner-Kersee, and Mike Powell suffer from this problem! It's impossible to avoid. Why? Because their takeoff foot pushing back at the board causes their bodies to rotate in the opposing direction. Worse still, their bodies will continue to rotate forward throughout their flight unless they do something about it. Their legs and feet then hit the sand prematurely and the distance jumped is greatly reduced. Novice jumpers who hold a bunched-up position in flight get themselves in great trouble because a tightly flexed position means that they also spin very quickly. As a result, a novice's body and feet quickly rotate down toward the sand and a poor distance is the result (see Figure 4.36).

To counteract unwanted forward rotation, an expert long jumper rotates the arms and legs in the same direction (i.e., forward) while in the air. Elite jumpers like Carl Lewis and Mike Powell, who have perfected the cycling action of a "hitch-kick," can stop their bodies from rotating forward and cause them to rotate in the opposing direction (see Figure 4.37). This change in rotation helps them achieve a good body position for landing and so increase the distance jumped.

Just how much reaction an athlete gets from rotating the arms and legs depends on how much angular momentum the athlete's body has at takeoff and how much the arm and leg actions introduce. Vigorous rotary actions with arms

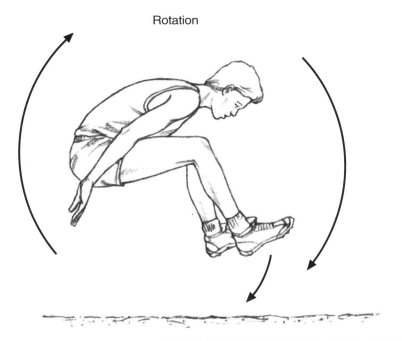

Fig. 4.36. In the air, a bunched position increases the long jumper's angular velocity and reduces the distance jumped.

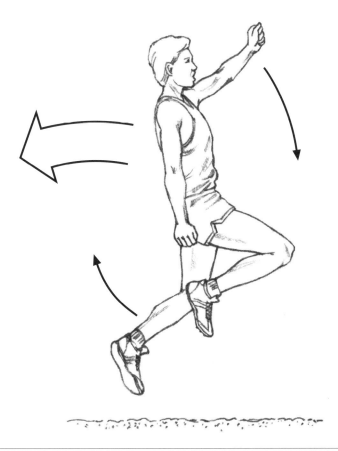

Fig. 4.37. Forward rotation of the arms and legs causes backward rotation of the long jumper's body.

and legs extended produce the most angular momentum. Look for expert long jumpers straightening out their legs and arms ahead of their bodies and then rotating them backward in an extended position. This has maximum effect on counteracting the forward rotation of the athlete's body.

A good place to see a desperate use of angular momentum is at your local swimming pool. Youngsters run and jump off the springboard. They don't expect the board to flip their feet upward to the rear and in horror they find themselves rotating in the air and heading for a belly flop. It's at this point that they introduce a wild flailing of the arms! These youngsters, uneducated in mechanics, are introducing angular momentum in the correct direction! They rotate their arms, and frequently their legs, in the same direction as the unwanted rotation that they have received from the springboard! Without knowing it, this action replicates in rough form the precise movements of an elite long jumper.

Transferring Angular Momentum Between Somersaults and Twists

Divers, gymnasts, and ski-aerialists frequently combine somersaults with twists. In these complex skills, athletes simultaneously somersault around their transverse axis (hip to hip) and twist around their long axis (feet to head). The most remarkable of the techniques used to combine somersaults with twists are those in which athletes begin by somersaulting with no twist apparent. Once in flight, the athletes perform a series of movements that cause the twist to occur. Then they perform a second series of movements that make the twist disappear. Let's look at diving and examine the mechanics of these actions.

At takeoff, divers push against the board to help get their body rotating and so generate angular momentum. As with long jumpers, the amount of angular momentum produced at takeoff remains virtually the same throughout the dive.

In flight the diver begins by rotating around the somersaulting axis (i.e., transverse or hip to hip). Then the diver performs a series of body actions that borrow or steal some angular momentum from the somersault to put into the twist. The diver now somersaults and twists. After somersaulting and twisting for the required number of revolutions, a second series of actions is performed. These remove the twist and the diver somersaults without twisting.

There is one dominant method for borrowing or stealing angular momentum from the somersault and placing it in the twist. This is called the **body tilt twist** technique.

The body tilt twist technique. This interesting technique requires that the diver's body be tilted away from its somersaulting axis so some angular momentum goes into the twisting axis. This is best understood by imagining the diver as a solid block somersaulting around the transverse (somersault) axis (see Figure 4.38, a, b, and c). The angular momentum that the diver has while in the flight is set at takeoff, so in Figure 4.38a, a specific amount of angular momentum is given to the block around its transverse axis. Suppose that during the somersaulting rotation, the block is made to tip over sideways so that it lies horizontally (see Figure 4.38b). Rotation continues, but the block now rotates around its longitudinal axis. In effect, the block's long axis has become its somersaulting axis.

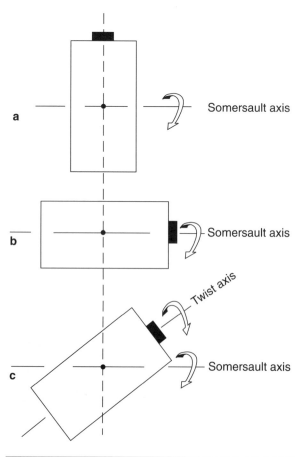

Fig. 4.38. Mechanics of body tilt twist.

Now let's tilt the block over just a few degrees (shown in Figure 4.38c) rather than all the way to horizontal. The block now twists and somersaults at the same time. Why? Because the angle of tilt forces some angular momentum into the twist axis (i.e., the block's long axis) and some remains in the original somersault axis. In addition, the rotary inertia (i.e., resistance) of the block around its twist axis is less than that around the somersault axis. The block twists faster than it somersaults. If the block is brought back from horizontal to its original position, the process is reversed. The twist disappears and all angular momentum goes back into the somersaulting axis.

Initiating body tilt. The principles described above indicate that if divers start a dive by somersaulting, they will somersault *and* twist if they tilt over slightly while in flight. But how do divers tilt themselves over while in the air? Here's how it occurs. When divers take off from the board they extend their arms sideways and upward (Figure 4.39a). In flight one arm swings downward and the other simultaneously swings upward (Figure 4.39b). Notice that even though one arm goes up and the other down, both arms rotate clockwise. The angular momentum generated by these clockwise arm actions causes the diver's body to react by rotating in a counterclockwise direction. A double arm swing of 90 degrees (one arm swung up 90 degrees and the other swung down 90 degrees) causes the body to tilt approximately 5 degrees from the vertical (see Figure 4.39b). Five degrees is sufficient for a diver to initiate a twist. Swinging the arms back reestablishes the original body position and eliminates the twist.

A common sequence for the combination of a somersault and twist using body tilt is as follows: The athlete begins the dive by initiating a somersault at takeoff. In flight, the diver raises one arm and lowers the other. The diver's body tilts over, which causes twists and somersaults to occur at the same time. When the diver returns the arms to their original positions, the twist is eliminated.

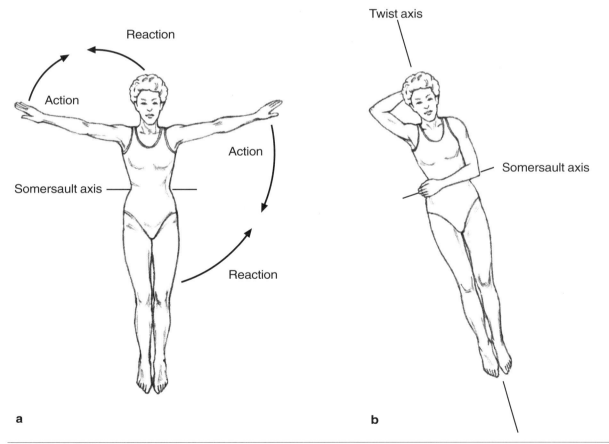

a
b

Fig. 4.39. Diver with arms outstretched (a) rotates around the somersault axis. When the diver raises one arm and lowers the other (b), the diver's body tilts. This causes some somersaulting momentum to be transferred to the twist axis.

The somersaulting action continues and is reduced to a minimum when the diver's body is fully extended for entry into the water.

Divers also are aware that the more body tilt they can establish, the more twists they can perform. What can be done to exaggerate the body tilt? After a half twist around the long axis is complete, the arm that was lowered is raised and wrapped to the rear of the head. The other arm, which had been raised, is lowered and pulled in tight across the waist. This repetitive arm action tilts the diver over farther causing twists to occur at an incredible rate. In this manner triple twisting somersaulting dives are made possible.

The cat twist technique. This technique is called the cat twist because a cat, like many other animals, performs the mechanics of this twisting technique naturally, without training or coaching. Experimentation has shown that if a cat is held inverted in a static position 2 to 3 ft from the ground and allowed to drop, the animal can initiate a twist in the air so that it can land safely on all fours. Figure 4.40, a-e, shows the cat falling. Notice the piked angle at the cat's midsection in Figure 4.40a. This is an important angle because it allows the cat to twist the upper body against the rotary inertia of the lower body and vice versa. The first move the cat makes is to establish visual contact with the ground. The cat pulls in the forelegs and turns the upper body toward the ground (see Figure 4.40, b-c). By pulling in the forelegs, the cat reduces the rotary inertia of the upper body in relation to its lower body, which has more rotary inertia because the rear legs are fully extended. Consequently the upper body, with its smaller rotary inertia, can be rotated through a large angle with minimal reaction in the opposing direction from the lower body. Once the cat sees the ground, the forelegs are extended ready for landing (see Figure 4.40d). This increases the rotary inertia of the upper body. The rear legs are pulled inward. This reduces the rotary inertia of the lower body and allows the lower body to rotate against the greater rotary inertia of the upper body. Once fully aligned the cat is ready to land safely (see Figure 4.40e).

The cat twist differs from the body tilt technique because it can be performed without having to borrow or steal angular momentum from a somersault. In other words an athlete does not have to be somersaulting to perform the cat twist action.

The cat twist always requires the athlete's body to have an angle or to be bent at the hips in some

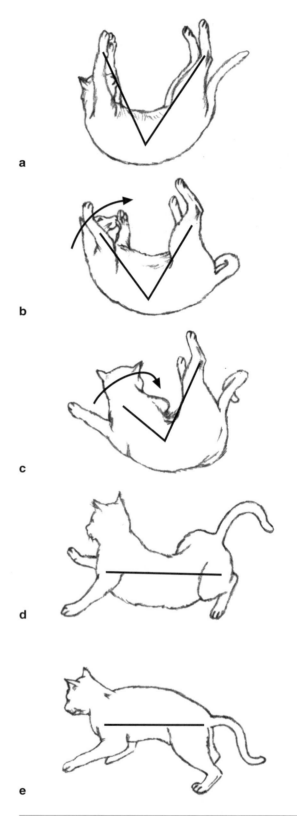

a

b

c

d

e

Fig. 4.40. Cat twist. The cat reduces the rotary inertia of the upper body and twists the upper body against the larger rotary inertia of the lower body. Notice the angle in the body in (a) to (c).

way. It doesn't matter what direction, flexion at the waist can be forward, backward, or sideways—they all work successfully! A 90-degree angle at the waist is preferable (i.e., with the upper body piked forward), but the cat twist can be performed with far less than 90 degrees. On the trampoline an elementary skill that employs the technique of the cat twist is the swivel hips.

The piked position used in the swivel hips also occurs in diving. Figure 4.41a shows a diver in a piked position with a right angle existing at the hips. In this position you can see that the mass of

the legs is a long way out relative to the long axis, which extends from the athlete's hips to the head. Figure 4.41b shows the athlete twisting the upper body against the greater rotary inertia of the legs. This is the basic principle of the cat twist. A twist is achieved by turning one part of the body that has reduced rotary inertia against another part that has much larger rotary inertia.

The cat twist is frequently used at the start of forward dives that contain somersaults and twists. In these dives the athlete will use both the cat twist and the body tilt technique. Figure 4.42, a-e,

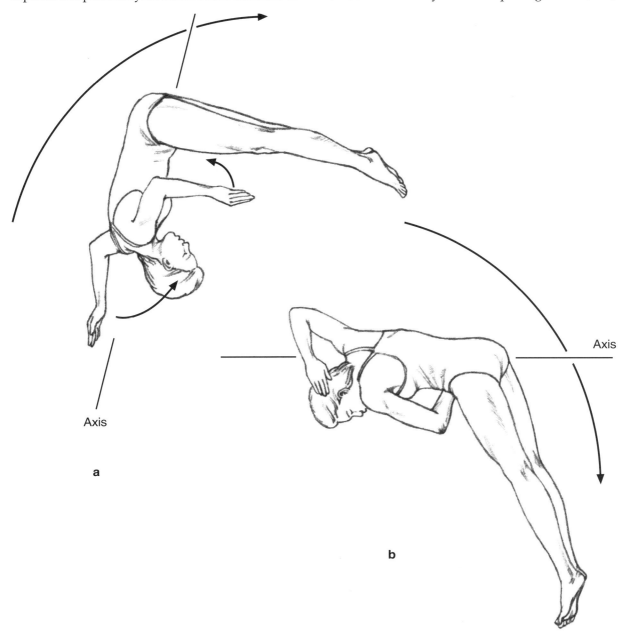

Fig. 4.41. Diver using a cat twist. The diver is in a piked position in (a) with a right angle at the hips. In (b), the diver twists the upper body against the greater rotary inertia of the legs.
Reprinted from Adrian and Cooper 1995.

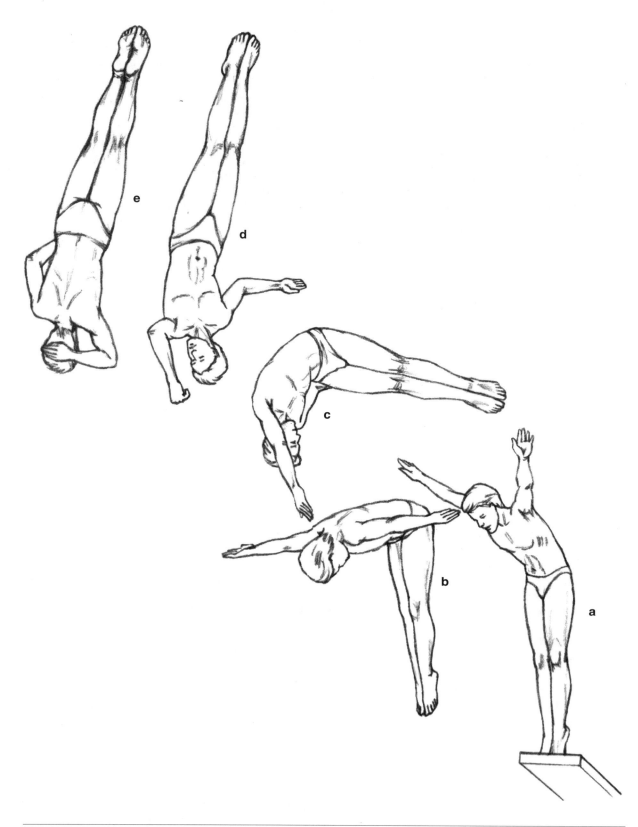

Fig. 4.42.   Diver simultaneously using the cat twist and body tilt twist technique after takeoff.

shows a diver taking off for a dive that will contain both somersaults and twists. Notice in Figure 4.42a the diver's arms are extended outward above the shoulders. Rotation around the transverse somersaulting axis is initiated at takeoff. Figure 4.42b shows the 90-degree pike required by the cat twist and the raising of one arm and the lowering of the other using the principles of the body tilt. Once the upper body is twisted against the inertia of the lower body, the angle at the waist is removed in Figure 4.42, d-e, to allow the twist to continue around the long axis of the diver's body.

The hula hoop twist technique. The hula hoop twisting technique is used by divers and especially by gymnasts. As in using the cat twist, a diver with zero angular momentum can initiate the hula hoop twist while in flight. In other words, a diver need not be rotating in any way to use the hula hoop twist.

You can recognize the hula hoop twist by the hula hoop action of the hips. Here's how the hula hoop twist works. If you are in the air and you rotate your hips in "Chubby Checker" fashion in a clockwise direction, your body will counteract this action by rotating *as a whole* in the opposite direction. A hula hoop action with the hips also makes the athlete's torso and legs follow cone-shaped pathways which are shown in Figure 4.43. Like the cat twist, the hula hoop twist is initiated by internal muscular force, and contact with the diving board is not required to get the twist started. Consequently, it can be initiated in midair: the faster the hula hoop action or the greater the amplitude of the circling upper and lower body parts, the faster the twist. The twist is also stopped when the hula hoop action ceases. In general, divers and gymnasts regard the large amplitude technique for increasing the rate of twist as less aesthetically pleasing than the faster action, and they try not to use it.

There are other twisting and somersaulting techniques used by divers and particularly by ski-aerialists. Unfortunately a discussion of these techniques is beyond the scope of this text. If you coach or intend to coach gymnastics, diving, skating, ski-aerials, trampoline, or any sport in which your athlete twists and turns in the air, be sure you understand the mechanics of the event and use proven safety techniques.

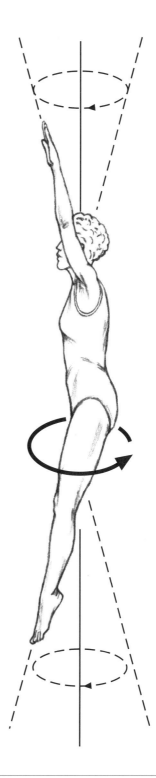

Fig. 4.43. Hula hoop twist. The broken arrows indicate the direction of rotation of the upper and lower body. The unbroken arrow indicates the direction of twist the diver's body makes as a whole.
Adapted from Rackham 1975.

SUMMARY

1. All rotational, turning, and swinging motions are forms of angular motion. Angular motion implies that an object or athlete rotates around an axis.

2. Motion in an athlete's body is predominantly rotational. Muscles pull on bones, and bones rotate at the joints.

3. Levers are simple machines that transmit mechanical energy. A lever incorporates a rigid object that rocks or rotates around an axis or fulcrum. Force is applied at one position on the lever, and a resistance applies its own force at another.

4. The two most important functions of a lever system are magnification of force and magnification of speed and distance.

5. There are three classes of levers. In a first class lever, the axis is positioned between the force and the resistance. First class levers can be made to magnify either force or speed and distance. In a second class lever, the resistance is positioned between the axis and the force. Second class levers magnify force at the expense of speed and distance. In a third class lever, the force is positioned between the axis and the resistance. Third class levers magnify speed and distance at the expense of force.

6. Third class levers predominate in the human body. Most muscles in the human body apply great force in order to move light resistances over large distances at great speed.

7. Levers produce a turning effect called torque. Torque is increased by magnifying the applied force and/or the distance from the axis of rotation that force is applied.

8. Angular velocity is synonymous with rate of spin. It refers to the angle/degrees/ revs completed in a particular time frame (e.g., sec) in a specific direction (e.g., clockwise or counterclockwise).

9. All objects that rotate or swing have an inward pulling force, called a centripetal force, that acts toward the axis of rotation. Centripetal force counteracts the inertial desire of objects to travel in a straight line.

10. A centripetal force has an equal and opposite force, called a centrifugal force, which acts away from the axis of rotation. Centripetal and centrifugal forces do not exist in the absence of rotation.

11. The inertia of all objects makes them resist rotation. Once forced to rotate, however, an object's inertia is expressed by its wanting to continue rotating.

12. Rotary inertia varies according to the mass of a spinning object and the way its mass is distributed. The greater the distance that mass is spread out from its axis of rotation, the greater the rotary inertia. The more compressed that mass is, relative to its axis of rotation, the greater the reduction of rotary inertia.

13. Angular momentum is the rotary equivalent of linear momentum: It describes the quantity of rotary momentum. The angular momentum of an object is determined by the product of its mass, angular velocity, and the distribution of its mass.

14. In flights of short duration (e.g., diving, long jump, gymnastics, and high jump), the amount of angular momentum generated by an athlete at takeoff remains the same for the duration of the flight: This indicates that the athlete's angular momentum is conserved.

15. When an athlete's angular momentum is conserved, the athlete's rate of spin (angular velocity) increases or decreases in relation to changes in the distribution of the athlete's mass. For example, the tighter the tuck, the greater the angular velocity.

16. In flight, an athlete's angular velocity increases or decreases in relation to the introduction of angular momentum by other body parts. Clockwise rotation of the athlete's body as a whole can be counteracted by introducing clockwise rotation in the athlete's arms and legs. The same principle applies to counterclockwise rotation.

17. Divers use combinations of the body tilt, cat twist, and hula hoop techniques to twist and somersault.

18. The body tilt technique of twisting requires athletes to be somersaulting *before* initiating the twist. This technique uses specific arm actions to tilt the body out of the somersaulting axis. The action transfers angular momentum from the somersault axis to the twist axis. Athletes then twist and somersault simultaneously. When the body tilt is removed, the twist is eliminated and the somersault continues.

19. The cat twist technique can be initiated in flight with zero angular momentum. No somersault need be initiated beforehand. This technique requires athletes to be piked or arched at the waist. The twist is achieved by twisting one part of the body that has reduced rotary inertia against another part that has larger rotary inertia.

20. The hula hoop twist technique can be initiated in flight with zero angular momentum. A hula hoop action at the waist causes cone-shaped movements to occur in the upper and lower body. If these actions are performed in one direction, the athlete's body as a whole rotates in the opposing direction.

REVIEW QUESTIONS

1. Two athletes perform strict biceps curls with 30 lb dumbbells. One athlete has much longer forearms. Why does the biceps curl demand more muscular force from the athlete with the longer forearms?

2. Swing a baseball bat forward and back around your body, noting how much effort you put into starting, stopping, and maneuvering the bat during the swing. Now hold the bat at the hitting end (i.e., the barrel end) and repeat the process. Why is it easier to start, stop, and maneuver the bat when held at the hitting end?

3. Perform a vertical jump and reach, swinging your arms upward as you take off. Now perform your jump and reach not with an arm *swing* but with both arms extended above your head. Explain the mechanical principles that account for the better jump performance when you swing your arms upward.

4. What components make up an athlete's angular momentum? Why is angular momentum conserved when divers, high jumpers, trampolinists, long jumpers, and gymnasts are in flight?

5. What equal and opposite reaction occurs when a flop jumper simultaneously lowers her legs and torso toward the pit as she arches over the bar?

6. What twisting techniques mentioned in the text do not require the athlete to be somersaulting before initiating a twist?

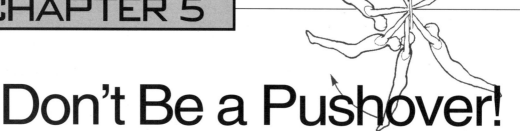

CHAPTER 5

Don't Be a Pushover!

When you finish reading this chapter, you should be able to explain

◼ the importance of balance, equilibrium, and stability in sport skills;

◼ how athletes make use of linear and rotary stability;

◼ the mechanical principles that determine different levels of linear and rotary stability;

◼ why some sport skills require minimal stability; and

◼ why the rotary stability of a spinning object is proportional to its angular momentum.

This chapter discusses the importance of equilibrium and stability in the performance of sport skills. You'll read how some sport skills require an athlete to maximize stability, and others require the athlete to reduce stability to minimum levels. You'll also see how an athlete's stability is related to mass, inertia, and momentum, and how an athlete's stability is always a battle of torques. The turning effect of one torque that disrupts an athlete's stability is battled by the turning effect of another torque applied by the athlete to regain equilibrium.

Many athletes naturally sense how to move and seem to know instinctively what they should do to maximize their stability. Unfortunately not all athletes are gifted this way. Young athletes, particularly those struggling to learn a new skill, use poor body positions that reduce the quality of their performances. They don't plant their feet properly when throwing, striking, or hitting, and they find that the reaction forces resulting from their actions cause them to stumble or fly in the opposite direction! These athletes don't assume efficient stances when checked, blocked, or challenged by an opponent. When they lose their balance, they don't make the best maneuvers to regain control quickly. If they want to move suddenly, they are unable to do so because their stances don't allow them to get off the mark quickly. All these examples are errors involving stability. Most of these errors are easy to correct if you teach the mechanical principles relating to stability, balance, and equilibrium. You'll read about these principles in this chapter.

Equilibrium, Balance, and Stability

Equilibrium and stability are two terms that are closely related but have different meanings. **Equilibrium** (or **balance**) implies coordination and control. An athlete with great balance can maintain a state of equilibrium and neutralize those forces that would disrupt her performance. When world champion gymnast Shannon Miller works flawlessly through a routine on the beam, she successfully counteracts the forces that would pull her off the beam. Shannon can maintain her equilibrium and so has great balance. Compare Shannon with Emmitt Smith of the Dallas Cowboys. Emmitt twists and turns, fends off tackles, and keeps driving for the line even though he's bombarded with tackles and checks from opponents. In spite of the great differences in their sports, Shannon and Emmitt both demonstrate great control and great balance.

Athletes must maintain their balance in skills in which there is little movement (e.g., Shannon performing a balance on the beam), and in skills that are highly dynamic (e.g., Emmitt driving for a touchdown). The enemy that athletes fight while trying to maintain balance can be any external force. Gravity, friction, air resistance, or force applied against them by opponents can destroy their performance.

Stability specifically relates to how much resistance athletes put up against having their equilibrium disturbed. The more stable an athlete, the more resistance the athlete generates against disruptive forces. An athlete can be in a state of equilibrium and be as stable as the Rock of Gibraltar. At the other extreme, an athlete can maintain equilibrium and yet be highly unstable. A 550 lb sumo wrestling champion like Hawaiian Salevaa

Atisnoe ("Konishiki") squatting low with both hands on the ground is obviously in a more stable position than a ballet star like Baryshnikov balancing on the tip of his toe. A child can produce enough force to push Baryshnikov off balance, but it's unlikely that the same force will do anything but bring a smile to Konishiki's face. Both Baryshnikov and Konishiki are in a state of equilibrium, but Konishiki is more stable.

Linear Stability

An athlete can have resistance against being moved in a particular direction and resistance against being stopped or having his or her direction changed once on the move. Both situations are types of **linear stability**. For example, Konishiki can resist being forced by his opponent in a particular direction. When Konishiki charges across the ring to slam into his opponent, his opponent then has to apply force to stop or change his direction.

If Konishiki weighed 600 lb instead of his top fighting weight of 556 lb, then he would need more strength to get himself moving. An opponent would require more force to move him from a stable position or change his direction once Konishiki charged across the ring. Konishiki's body weight is related to his mass, and his mass is synonymous with how much inertia he has. Consequently, the more massive Konishiki becomes, the more inertia he has—and the more stability he has too. So linear stability is directly related to mass, inertia, and also Konishiki's mass when it's on the move. Increase any of these factors and stability increases too. Sumo wrestlers are well aware of this fact. It's for this reason that they are forever stuffing themselves with food and trying to put on weight!

Whether athletes want to have great linear stability depends on the demands of the skill. In the Olympic Games, rowers want to maintain the straightest course possible. To do this they try to eliminate any forces that might shift them off course. A U.S. heavyweight rowing eight powering toward the finish has tremendous linear stability. Collectively, the eight rowers and their shell form a huge mass. The long, narrow shape of their shell coupled with their rowing actions propel them at high speed in a straight line. The opposition trying to push them off their straight line course is predominately from wind, waves, and friction generated by moving through the air and water.

Surfers, skaters, and slalom skiers differ from the rowing eight because these athletes are particularly interested in sudden directional changes. They will want some linear stability, but they don't want to keep going in a straight line when it's necessary to make tight turns. So athletes who want to shift and turn quickly avoid tipping the scales like a sumo wrestler. Imagine world champion slalom skier Alberto Tomba trying to maneuver 500 lb of body weight through a series of tight turns! It's no different for squash players, badminton players, and goal keepers in soccer. Tremendous body mass means too much stability, and it can be a liability in skills in which high speed reactions are the order of the day.

Linear Stability and Friction

The more friction that acts on an athlete, the more difficult it is to get the athlete moving. A massive wrestler like U.S. Olympic heavyweight champion Bruce Baumgartner lying in a defensive position on a wrestling mat is very difficult to move. Gravity pulls his huge mass down tight onto the mat and as a result he becomes "glued" to the mat! If, during a competition, Bruce was able to increase his weight (e.g., from 280 lb to 300 lb), then the additional pressure from his extra body mass would press him down onto the mat even more, and increase friction that much more too! You can see why Bruce's opponent must have phenomenal strength and plenty of energy if he wants to pull or push Bruce across the mat.

Compare this scenario with a speed skater like Dan Jansen. Dan is much lighter than Bruce Baumgartner and the frictional differences between a wrestling mat and slick ice are obvious! The slightest thrust overcomes the friction of Dan's blades on the ice and he glides effortlessly as a result. His linear stability in this situation is minimal; Bruce Baumgartner's linear stability is maximal.

Whatever the type of surface, a massive athlete like Bruce Baumgartner presses down onto the ground or a supporting surface more than a speed skater like Dan Jansen, or a lightweight gymnast like Shannon Miller. In fact, Bruce will press down on the ground more than an opponent who is only a few ounces lighter! In football, the pressure produced by the mass of a huge lineman pressing down on the earth generates more friction between his cleats and the turf than that produced by a lightweight running back. This gives the lineman better traction than the running back. (Of course, the lineman has more mass and inertia than a running back, so although he may have more traction, he doesn't have a running back's maneuverability!) An opponent must overcome the lineman's friction with the turf if he wants to block him out of a play.

Rotary Stability

Rotary stability is the resistance of an athlete or an object against being tilted, tipped over, upended, or spun around in a circle. However, if an athlete or an object (e.g., a discus) is spun around, then rotary stability can also describe the ability of the athlete and the discus to keep spinning. Let's look at the principles that help an athlete avoid falling, being tipped over, upended, or spun around. These principles are universal in sport and extremely important.

The effort that an athlete uses to maintain balance varies from sport to sport. An elite sprinter is not concerned with balance and stability during a 100 m race, and a top-class basketball player doesn't expect to fall over when bringing the ball up court. However there are other sports in which the athlete must actively work to maintain their balance and equilibrium. For example, in the sport of judo, the athletes battle to maintain their balance and must maneuver out of the way of their opponent's leg sweeps to avoid being thrown. American weight lifter and world record holder Karyn Marshall fights to hold a 275 lb barbell above her head. Aussie world champion sprint cyclist Gary Niewand works hard to balance on his bike as he plays cat and mouse with his opponent at the start of a sprint race. These athletes are maintaining their rotary stability. When they have excellent rotary stability, they can resist the destabilizing and upending effect of a powerful torque, or turning effect, applied against them. The more stable they are, the more torque is necessary to upset their balance. Let's see how this battle of torques gets started.

The destabilizing effect of a torque that upsets an athlete's balance can come from any external source. It could be generated by gravity, air resistance, an opponent, or by a combination of forces. The axis around which athletes rotate when a torque is applied against them can be anyplace on their bodies. Most frequently, it's their feet, but it can just as well be their shoulders, hips, or their hands. On the beam, if Shannon Miller loses her balance, the axis of rotation will be where her body contacts the beam. It can be the ball of one foot during a pirouette or her hands during a handstand. In a hip throw in judo, the point of rotation is where the athlete's body contacts the opponent's hip. If Carl Lewis stumbles during a lunge for the tape, the point of rotation is likely to be his spikes where they contact the track.

Torque Versus Torque

When an elite gymnast performs an extremely difficult one-handed handstand, she is in a highly unstable state of equilibrium. She fights hard to maintain this delicate state of equilibrium. If she allows her body to shift the slightest distance out of balance, a turning effect (or torque) occurs as she starts to rotate. The earth pulls at her center of gravity. The axis of rotation will be her hand on the floor or on the apparatus. The farther she shifts out of a balanced position, the greater the turning effect. In a one-handed balance, a gymnast has to use the strength in her supporting hand and forearm (plus other muscles in her body) to counter a shift out of a balanced position. She does this by producing an opposing torque. If the turning effect of this torque is sufficient, it will rotate the gymnast in the opposite direction until she regains a state of balance. But if she allows her center of gravity to shift too great a distance from its correct position (which is directly above the supporting hand), she may not have the strength to pull herself back to a balanced position. Gravity then wins this battle of torque and the gymnast collapses out of the balance. Figure 5.1 shows a gymnast who has allowed her center of gravity to shift too far to the left. The greater this distance (d) the greater the torque produced by gravity.

Compare a gymnast balancing in a one-handed handstand to that of the defending wrestler shown in Figure 5.2. Both are in a state of equi-

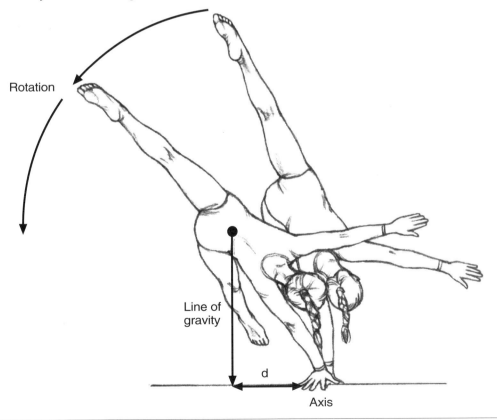

Fig. 5.1. When the center of gravity is no longer above the supporting base, gravity applies a destabilizing torque. The greater the distance (d) of the line of gravity from the axis, the greater the torque produced by gravity.

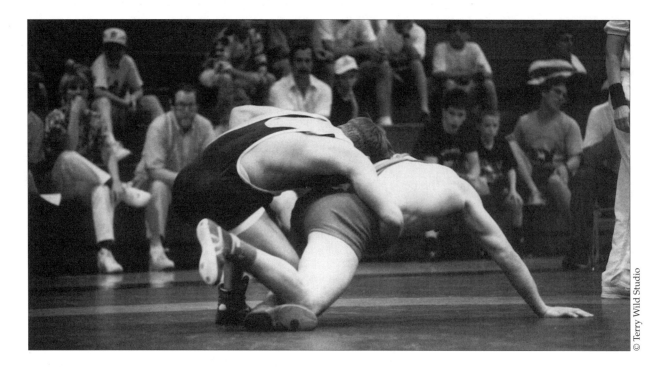

Fig. 5.2. By pulling the defending wrestler's hand off the floor, the attacker has reduced the area of the defender's supporting base, although he is still relatively stable.

librium. But it's easy to see that the wrestler's position on the mat is far more stable. Even if the wrestler maintained the same stance (without shifting or performing any additional maneuvers), the attacking wrestler must apply tremendous torque to lift and rotate him out of this defensive position.

Figure 5.3 shows another example from wrestling. This illustration shows how rotary stability is a war of torque. The torque applied by the attacker (i.e., force × force arm) competes against the torque (i.e., resistance × resistance arm) generated in the opposing direction by the defending wrestler. In this situation the defending wrestler's body weight acts as the resistance and his hand is the axis of rotation. The attacker tries to increase the turning effect he's applying to his opponent by increasing the force he's applying and the length of the force arm he's using. The defending wrestler obviously cannot increase his body weight during a wrestling match! But what he tries to do is keep his resistance arm as long as possible. In Figure 5.3 you can see that the defending wrestler could lengthen his resistance arm by shifting his hand on the mat farther from his opponent! So what we have here is a battle of

torque (i.e., force × force arm fighting against resistance × resistance arm).

Let's stay with the sport of wrestling and imagine heavyweight Bruce Baumgartner lying face down and spread-eagled on the mat. Every time the opponent grabs Bruce's arm or leg to turn him over, Bruce immediately shifts his body so the attacker never gets into a position that gives him good leverage. This situation would be like using a crowbar to raise a rock and finding that the rock keeps moving and never lets you get into a position where you can use the crowbar to advantage!

Compare this situation with that of a gymnast balancing on one foot on the beam (see Figure 5.4). Bruce does everything possible to maximize his rotary stability. He is massive, his center of gravity cannot be positioned any lower to the ground, and he shifts his mass and spreads his arms and legs to counteract the torque applied by his attacker. The gymnast has her center of gravity high above the beam, and to make matters worse, she is balancing on one foot! Both the gymnast and Bruce successfully maintain their equilibrium. The gymnast has minimal rotary stability because it takes very little force and

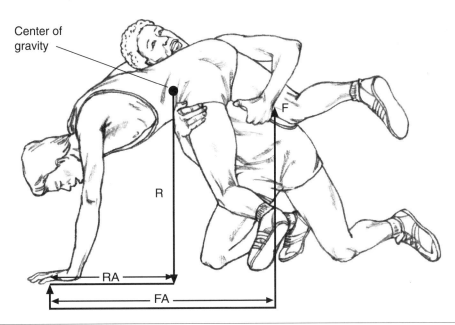

Fig. 5.3. Wrestling is a battle of torque. The attacker's force (F) × force arm (FA) competes against the defender's resistance (R) × resistance arm (RA).

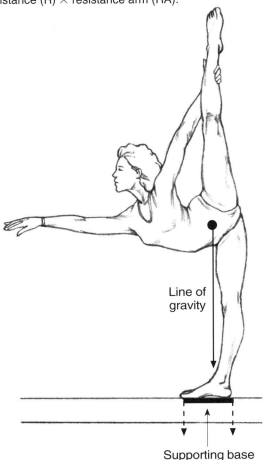

Fig. 5.4. Gymnast's supporting base is the area covered by the foot on the beam. The line of gravity falls within the area of the base.

torque to destabilize her. Bruce constantly positions himself to have maximum rotary stability.

Factors Determining Rotary Stability

The conditions that give the gymnast minimal stability and Bruce Baumgartner maximal stability are clues to the mechanical principles that determine rotary stability. These principles are important because they occur in every sport skill. Let's look at them one at a time and see how they affect an athlete's performance.

• **Athletes increase their stability when they increase the size of their base of support.** This means that the bigger an athlete's base of support the greater is the athlete's stability. A **base of support** most commonly refers to the area on the ground enclosed by the points of contact of the athlete's body. We use the words "most commonly" here because a base is not always below the athlete. Anything that provides resistance against forces exerted by the athlete can become a base. If a student in an aerobics class leans against the wall in a calf-stretching exercise, she has a base that includes the wall and the ground. A gymnast hanging from one of the uneven bars has a base that is a bar and happens to be overhead.

What do we mean by "area" when we talk of the base of support? When a gymnast balances on one foot on the beam, she uses the area of her foot as a base of support. If she places her other foot onto the beam, her base of support now stretches from one foot to the other. With two feet on the beam the gymnast is more stable than when on one foot. As you can guess, with two feet on the beam, her stability is better forward and backward than it is from the side. It's more difficult to shove the gymnast off the beam if you push from the front or the back, than if you push from the side. Returning to Figure 5.2, the defensive wrestler has a triangular base that stretches from his hand on the mat to his knees. His opponent has pulled one of the defending wrestler's hands off the mat and has reduced the size of his base of support. In Figure 5.3 the defending wrestler's base of support stretches from the single hand on the mat to where he contacts his opponent. Because his opponent is trying to turn him over onto his shoulders for a pin, it's obvious that an opponent can hardly be considered a stable base of support!

You can see from these examples that stability is directly related to the size of the supporting base. Make your base as big as possible and you are more stable. A gymnast in a one-handed handstand has a base that is solely the area of her hand. If a gymnast lowers to a headstand, the base now becomes the triangular shape that runs from the head to the hands (see Figure 5.5). When Bruce Baumgartner lies flat on the mat and spreads out his legs and arms as wide as possible, he covers a huge area that runs from his fingertips to his feet. As far as the size of his base is concerned, Bruce has made himself maximally stable. If you're a wrestler you'll use this position when you're defending and also when you're attacking. If you're attacking and you want to hold your opponent in a particular position and stop him from moving, maximize your stability just as you would if you were defending. By maximizing your stability you make it difficult for your opponent to mount a counterattack!

• **Athletes increase their stability when their line of gravity falls within the perimeter of their base of support.** An athlete maintains balance as long as a vertical line passing through the athlete's center of gravity falls inside the perimeter of the base of support. The closer to the center of the base this **line of gravity** falls (i.e., like a plumb line), the more stable the athlete becomes.

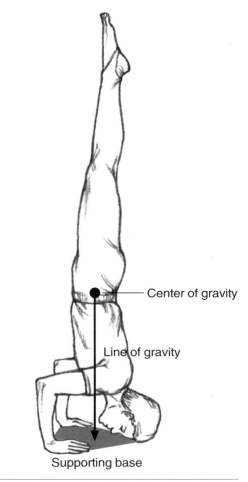

Fig. 5.5. In a headstand, the supporting base is the triangular area from the head to the hands.

Conversely, the closer to the edge of the base the line of gravity falls, the more unstable the athlete becomes. The larger the base, the easier it is for an athlete to make sure that this vertical line falls within the base.

To understand how the position of the line of gravity relates to stability, let's start with a famous tourist attraction—the Leaning Tower of Pisa in Italy. The tower has been closed to tourists since 1900 because its line of gravity had been getting dangerously close to the edge of its base. The more it leans, the more the line of gravity shifts toward the edge, and the more unstable it becomes. If the tower's line of gravity should ever pass outside its base, then gravity could produce a torque with more turning effect than what would keep the tower upright. So it's essential for the stability of the tower that its line of gravity remains within the perimeter of the base. There are several methods that can make the tower more stable. Engineers could follow our first principle, which is to widen the base of the tower. But this action would spoil the tower's architectural beauty. Other methods for stabilizing the tower are being carried out, such as adding almost 700 tons of lead ingots to its base and on the side opposing the direction of lean!

Unlike the Leaning Tower of Pisa and other inanimate objects, living beings can maneuver and shift position, and in this way keep their line of gravity above their base. If an athlete's base is small there's little leeway for error. If you are balancing above a very small base and allow your center of gravity to shift the slightest distance, then you've given gravity a chance to apply a torque that you may not be able to counteract. That's one reason a gymnast's one-handed handstand is such a phenomenal feat requiring tremendous strength and control! The base of support is solely the area covered by the athlete's supporting hand. The athlete's center of gravity cannot shift more than an inch from directly above the supporting hand. So all the athlete's muscles work to hold the center of gravity in position.

In contrast to the one-handed handstand is a wrestler's spread-eagled defensive position. Assuming that the wrestler's center of gravity is close to his navel, the line of his center of gravity would have to shift several feet in any direction before it would get anywhere near the perimeter of his base! It's no wonder that wrestlers use this position so often.

You must not think that athletes always want to have their line of gravity continuously within the base. When you walk or run, you take a series of steps forward. With each leg swing your center of gravity shifts forward and outside of your base and you shift from a stable to an unstable position. When you put your foot down at the end of the step, your center of gravity is between your feet and you are in a stable position again (see Figure 5.6). When Olympic champions Gail Devers or Carl Lewis sprint, they go from one unstable position to another as they drive themselves along the track. One moment their line of gravity is outside their supporting base, the next instant it is inside again. This happens all the way down the track. The same situation occurs when hockey players like Wayne Gretzky and Eric Lindros skate down the ice.

When runners, skaters, cyclists, and slalom skiers go around a curve, they lean into the curve. Here you have an example of dynamic equilibrium, or equilibrium while on the move. If they

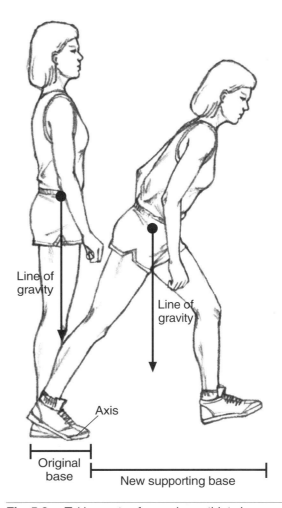

Fig. 5.6. Taking a step forward, an athlete becomes unstable, restabilizing when both feet again contact the ground.

came to a sudden stop in the middle of the curve, they would fall. As they lean into the curve the athletes' line of gravity no longer falls within their supporting base. The faster they move and the tighter the curve, the more they lean inward and the farther their center of gravity (and the line of their center of gravity) shifts into the curve. The correct amount of lean balances the forces acting into the curve with those acting outward (see Figure 5.7).

• **Athletes increase their stability when they lower their center of gravity.** An athlete whose center of gravity is high off her base of support is less stable than an athlete whose center of gravity is lower. So great running backs tend to be shorter than other football players, and run low to the ground. In this way they are more stable

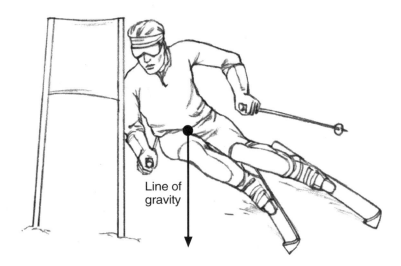

Line of gravity

Fig. 5.7. An athlete rounding a curve is in a state of dynamic equilibrium. Forces acting into the curve balance those acting outward.

and maintain their balance better than taller athletes.

To understand how stability relates to the height of an athlete's center of gravity, let's have an athlete using the same size base first stand erect and then crouch down. In both positions we'll tip the athlete sideways the same angle. Notice in Figure 5.8 that for the same angle of tilt, the line of the athlete's center of gravity shifts beyond the edge of the supporting base when the athlete is standing erect. When the athlete is crouching or squatting down the line of gravity is still within the base. This means that if other stability variables remain the same, the lower the athlete's center of gravity, the more stable the athlete becomes.

The principle of lowering the center of gravity to increase stability is one reason athletes crouch or lie flat on the mat when they are defending in combatives. Athletes in wrestling and judo not only lower their center of gravity but also widen their base of support. This increases their stability twofold, making it more difficult for an opponent to turn them over. Ski jumpers know that they lose points if they stagger on landing. Lowering their center of gravity as they land helps them to maintain their equilibrium. Kayakers who are tall and have most of their weight in their upper bodies have a high center of gravity. They are less stable than shorter athletes or athletes who have most of their weight in their hips and seat. (Taller kayakers can counteract this problem by using a kayak that has a wider beam, which widens their base of support.)

Weight lifting gives us many examples of reduction in stability when the center of gravity is elevated. The more weight that a weight lifter

Reduce Potential Energy and You Increase Stability

A skateboarder at the top of a ramp has plenty of potential energy. As the athlete accelerates down the ramp, potential energy is exchanged for kinetic energy, and on the way up the other side, kinetic energy becomes potential energy again. If the athlete didn't use muscular force to pump the action, the athlete would roll back and forth and end up at the bottom of the ramp in a state of stable equilibrium with no potential or kinetic energy. Reduce potential energy, and you move your center of gravity closer to the surface of the earth. In this way you increase your stability.

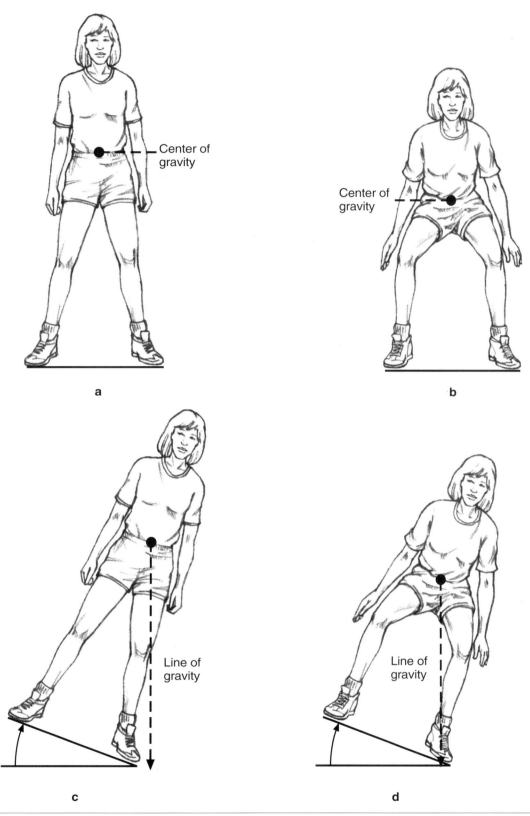

Fig. 5.8. When all else is equal, the higher the center of gravity, the less stable the state of equilibrium. An athlete stands erect (a) and crouches (b). For the same angle of sideway tilt, the line of the athlete's center of gravity shifts beyond the edge of the supporting base when the athlete is standing erect (c), but remains within the base when the athlete is crouching or squatting (d).

hoists and the longer the athlete's arms, the higher is the combined center of gravity of athlete and barbell. The line of this common center of gravity must stay centralized above a long but narrow base. If the athlete allows the barbell to shift out of line, he must reposition his base and fight with his shoulder muscles to bring the barbell back in line so it's centralized above his base. Figure 5.9 shows the final position in a clean and jerk. Stability in this position is better forward and backward because the base is large in that direction. But the base is narrow side to side. This means that even small sideways movements by the athlete can shift the common line of gravity of athlete and barbell outside the periphery of the athlete's base. The number of times that you see a weight lifter successfully raise a barbell to arm's length above the head, only to stagger and lose control, is an indication of the precarious stability of this position.

• **Athletes who increase their body mass increase their stability.** This principle simply says that if all other factors relating to stability are equal, a heavier and more massive athlete is more stable than one with less body mass. This is why there are weight divisions in combative sports.

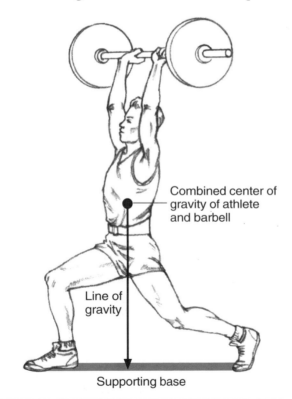

Combined center of gravity of athlete and barbell

Line of gravity

Supporting base

Fig. 5.9. In a clean and jerk, the common center of gravity of both the weight lifter and bar must be centralized above the supporting base.

What hope would multiple World and Olympic featherweight champion John Smith have (at 130 lb) trying to lift and rotate super-heavyweight Bruce Baumgartner at close to 300 lb?

The value of body mass in combatives is duplicated in football where huge linemen must maintain their positions in face of whatever is thrown against them. The heavier they are, the more force (and torque) it takes to throw them off balance and to knock them out of position. It's for this reason that they weigh close to 300 lb. There are no weight divisions in football like there are in Olympic wrestling.

In all sport skills, a heavier athlete who is out of control and has lost equilibrium must exert more muscular force to regain balance than a lighter athlete. If heavier athletes don't have the muscular strength, their extra body mass becomes a disadvantage rather than an advantage. Judo practitioners (judoka) try to use their opponent's body weight, and if their opponents are on the move, to make full use of their opponent's momentum! Judoka know that it's inefficient and exhausting to try to stop an opponent's push and afterward set up rotation in the opposing direction. Better to step out of the way, trip the opponent so there's an axis of rotation, and add your torque to that of gravity as your opponent rotates toward the mat! Smaller sumo wrestlers who try to dethrone Hawaiian-American champion Konishiki attempt the same maneuvers. It's obviously a good idea to get out of the way when 550 lb is charging at you. If you're one of Konishiki's opponents, you trip him and destabilize him as he rushes by! You then add your own force to that of gravity to drive him to the dirt floor, or more satisfying, to heave him among the spectators!

• **Athletes increase their stability when they extend their base in the direction of an oncoming force.** Whatever type of base is used, stability is increased if the athlete's supporting base is enlarged in the direction of an oncoming force. This force can be external and come from an opponent, or it can be internal and applied by an athlete, such as in throwing or hitting. Let's look at the first of these. If running back Emmitt Smith wants to maintain stability and continue running when hit by an opponent, he must consider the force of the hit and the direction it's coming from. To maintain stability and stay upright, Emmitt widens his base in the direction of the applied force. If the hit is coming from the front, he widens his base from front to back. If it comes from the side, he widens his base in that direction. Naturally, Emmitt is going to lean into the hit as well. We explain the mechanical principles of leaning into the hit later in this chapter.

The second application of this principle applies to situations in which athletes apply force in a particular direction. If you watch throwers, pitchers, and hitters, you'll notice that they widen their base in the direction they are applying force. Why do this? It gives them a stable base and it allows them to apply force over a considerable distance without losing balance. If they didn't do this, they'd be thrown in the opposite direction. It doesn't matter whether you're blasting a home run, or hurling a fastball, or just having fun in a pickup softball game, the same principles apply (see Figure 5.10).

The size of the base that an athlete uses in the conditions described above depends on how much force is applied. Imagine tossing a

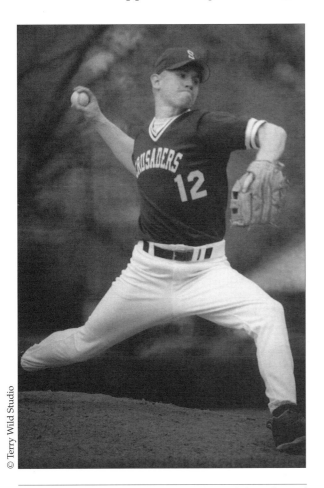

© Terry Wild Studio

Fig. 5.10. An athlete's supporting base is lengthened in the direction in which force is applied (i.e., in the direction of the pitch).

superlight table tennis ball a few yards. You could do this without any trouble while balancing on one foot. The table tennis ball has very little weight (i.e., mass) and in this situation is given very little velocity. Now try throwing a huge medicine ball as far as possible while balancing on one foot. You'll find that as the medicine ball goes one direction you get pushed in the opposite direction! (By the way, did you guess that throwing the medicine ball is the action, and you moving in the opposite direction is the reaction?)

Let's compare catching the table tennis ball lobbed gently toward you with catching a heavy object (like the medicine ball) traveling at a much higher velocity. You could easily catch the table tennis ball while balancing on one foot. Its momentum would be minimal and you could maintain your balance on one foot without any trouble. The medicine ball presents a different situation. If you want to maintain your stability and not have the medicine ball knock you over, you must have a wide stance with both feet well planted on the ground. You reach toward the ball and extend your stance in the direction that the medicine ball is approaching. The more massive the ball and the greater its velocity, the more stable must be your stance.

• **Athletes increase their stability when they move their line of gravity toward an oncoming force.** This principle is directly related to the one we've just been discussing. It says to an athlete: "Widen your base in the direction of an oncoming force, and move your center of gravity toward the force." Running backs purposely lean into tackles and blocks. Legendary ice hockey players like Bobby Orr, Gordie Howe, and Bobby Hull were masters at this art! These athletes shifted their center of gravity toward their opponents. This action not only stabilized them but forced their opponents to expend energy pushing them back into a more stable position! Think how easy it would be to knock over an opponent if you tackled from the front and your opponent was already leaning backward! On the other hand, if your opponent leans into your tackle, you have to push much farther before your opponent is off balance. The extra distance will also provide time for your opponent to make additional defensive maneuvers such as spinning out of the way.

The principle of shifting your center of gravity toward an oncoming force applies not only in tackles and checks but also when catching a heavy object like a medicine ball. Widen your base and shift your center of gravity toward the oncoming medicine ball. In this way you are stable when you catch the ball, and equally important, you give yourself lots of time to apply force to slow down the medicine ball. Do you recognize that "lots of time to apply force" is an expression of impulse used for stopping (i.e., a moderate force applied over a large time frame)? It's the moderate force applied over a long time frame that allows you to bring the ball comfortably to a stop.

An important difference exists when you are an athlete *applying force* rather than receiving it in a tackle. In this case lengthen your base in the direction of the applied force, but start your application of force with the line of your center of gravity close to, or even outside, the *rear* of your base. All good javelin throwers start their throw from a position where they are leaning backward, with their center of gravity well behind their base of support. Then in the follow-through they finish with their center of gravity way beyond the front edge of their base. In this way they apply force over the longest possible distance. This is another expression of impulse in action (see Figure 5.11).

In combatives like wrestling and judo, it's important that athletes be aware of the dangers inherent in shifting their center of gravity too close to the perimeter of their base. Imagine you're in a judo competition. You're pushing and leaning into your opponent and the opponent is doing the same to you. Your center of gravity is close to the front edge of your base. Suddenly your opponent stops pushing and instead pulls hard. Now there's

no resistance for you to push against and the force of your own push has suddenly been increased by the addition of your opponent's pull. You find that your center of gravity is outside your base and that you're totally unstable.

If you can sense that a push is about to change into a pull, immediately shift your center of gravity in the opposing direction and widen your base to get stable again. This cat and mouse game involving the positioning of the athlete's center of gravity is the essence of judo. One instant you're stable, the next instant you're rotating around an axis set up by a leg sweep from your opponent.

How All Principles of Rotary Stability Are Interrelated

Remember that all the factors that control rotary stability are closely interrelated. It's no good if an athlete makes one maneuver to increase stability if all the other factors controlling stability aren't satisfied as well. For example, if an athlete widens her base of support, she must widen it in the direction of an applied force. A rugby player can widen her base toward a tackle coming from the right, but if her line of the center of gravity stays close to the left edge of her base, she will easily be knocked over and beaten by the tackle. You know that a giant super-heavyweight is more stable than a lighter athlete, but extra body weight is of little use if this super-heavyweight uses a narrow base and stands with his center of grav-

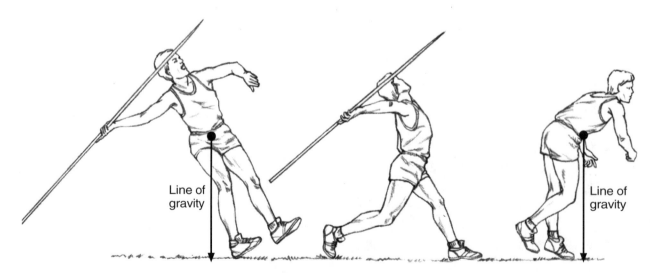

Line of gravity

Line of gravity

Fig. 5.11. In the javelin throw, the athlete's center of gravity begins to the rear of the supporting base and ends in front of the thrower's base.

ity high and close to the edge of his base. Likewise, an athlete who lowers her center of gravity improves her stability, but this action is only valuable if her line of gravity is within her base. So remember that all the principles of stability are related and each depends upon the other. Just obeying one principle of stability isn't good enough. You have to obey as many as possible.

Skills That Require Minimal Stability

We've been talking at length about maximizing stability. Are there skills in which athletes want to minimize their stability? Yes! Examples occur during the explosive acceleration of athletes like ice hockey star Pavel Bure and basketball great Michael Jordan. It also occurs during the swimming starts of Janet Evans and the sprint starts of Olympic champion Linford Christie. In a sprint start, a sprinter like Linford aims to get out of the blocks as fast as possible. On the "get set" command, he shifts his line of gravity forward so that it is very close to his hand positions on the track (see Figure 5.12). This highly unstable position satisfies two requirements. It extends Linford's legs into a powerful thrusting stance. Second, it puts Linford into a position that requires minimum force to thrust him in the required direction, toward the finishing line.

In sport skills in which sudden direction changes occur, athletes want to be able to shift quickly in any direction. The set position in Linford's sprint start is excellent for sudden and fast movement toward the finish in a 100 m race. But you'd be highly amused if you saw Pete Sampras or Steffi Graf using a sprinter's set position when they're waiting to receive a serve. Linford's set position might be good for a sudden move in one direction, but it's useless for moving quickly in other directions! Volleyball players receiving a serve and soccer goalkeepers defending the goal all need to be quick off the mark no matter what direction. They cannot guarantee the direction, velocity, or spin of the ball, and they don't want to commit themselves too early. Consequently, these athletes will use a fairly small base with their line of gravity centralized. In this way it takes only a split second to shift their center of gravity in the direction they want to move. They can react quickly and move fast in any direction.

Rotary Stability When Twisting, Turning, or Spinning

When an object or an athlete is rotating, swinging, or turning, their rotary stability is dependent upon their angular momentum. The more angular momentum, the more stability. From chapter

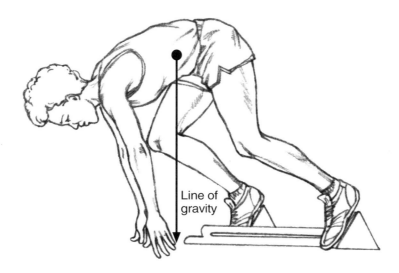

Fig. 5.12. In a sprint start, the athlete's line of gravity is shifted close to the forward edge of the supporting base.

A Tightrope Walker's Pole Increases Stability

Circus stars like the Great Wallendas have built a seven-person pyramid balancing on a single high wire. In 1974 tightrope walker Phillipe Petit of France walked across a high wire strung between the towers of the World Trade Center. Why are these daredevil performers more stable when they use a long pole, and why are they even more stable when the pole is really long, curved downward, and weighted at either end? Answer: A pole that curves downward lowers the center of gravity of performer and pole combined. If weights are added at the ends of the pole, it lowers the center of gravity even farther. In addition, the longer the weighted pole the greater rotary inertia and its resistance against rotation. This characteristic helps stop the performer from tipping sideways and falling off the wire. Without a long, curved, weighted pole, tightrope walkers would have a tough time maintaining balance!

4 you'll remember that angular momentum is determined by how fast an object rotates (i.e., its angular velocity), how massive it is, and how its mass is spread out or compressed relative to its axis of rotation. How does this type of rotary stability show up in sport? Here are some examples: A man's discus at 4 lb 6 oz (2 kg) is twice as massive as a woman's discus, and it's over 2 in. larger in diameter. If all other factors are equal, a man's discus (by virtue of its greater mass and size) will battle the destabilizing effect of wind better than a woman's discus.

Similar to a discus, a football will remain more stable in flight when it spins. The more spin, the greater the angular momentum of the football and the greater its stability. In this situation you're increasing angular momentum by increasing the ball's angular velocity, or spin. You're not changing it's mass or the distribution of its mass. When John Elway or Warren Moon rifle a pass to a receiver, the ball simulates the flight characteristics of a bullet. The high spin around the ball's long axis gives the ball what is called "gyroscopic stability" (i.e., stability resulting from spin). This helps the ball to resist destabilizing forces that air currents and air resistance produce. Without the spin, the ball will tumble and flutter in the air. Its flight will not be true nor will it travel as far. The same situation will occur to a discus thrown without spin.

Cyclists who use aerodynamic disc wheels on their bikes to improve their streamlining find that they cannot accelerate as well as when they use spoked wheels. Disc wheels tend to be heavier and so have more inertia. Once spinning, the wheels want to keep rotating like a flywheel on an engine. The wheels' desire to keep spinning is an expression of their rotary stability as well as their rotary inertia.

Unfortunately, a problem occurs when cyclists use discs on front and back wheels. Even though spinning disc wheels have more stability, they also present a large surface area, and a strong crosswind can shove a cyclist right off the road. Unless there's no wind or they're cycling in a wind-protected velodrome, cyclists commonly use a disc only on the back wheel. In this way they have no problem with wind upsetting their steering!

SUMMARY

1. Balance is synonymous with equilibrium. A well-balanced athlete can counteract those forces that might disrupt her equilibrium.

2. Stability implies resistance against the loss of equilibrium. There are two types of stability: linear and rotary stability.

3. At rest, an athlete's linear stability is proportional to his mass and the frictional forces occurring between the athlete and any supporting surfaces. While moving, an athlete's linear stability is directly related to momentum. The more massive the athlete and the faster his movements, the greater the athlete's linear stability.

4. Rotary stability implies resistance against being tipped over and upended. It also indicates resistance of a rotating object or athlete against a reduction in rate of spin.

5. An athlete's resistance against being tipped over or upended increases if (a) the area of her supporting base is enlarged, (b) the athlete's line of gravity falls within the boundaries of her supporting base, (c) the athlete lowers her center of gravity, (d) she increases her body mass, (e) the athlete's supporting base extends toward an oncoming force, or (f) her line of gravity shifts toward an oncoming force.

6. Some sport skills require minimal stability. Sprinters in the set position shift their lines of gravity toward the edge of their supporting bases and in the direction they will race. Athletes who need to move quickly in any direction keep their supporting bases relatively small and centralize their lines of gravity.

7. In situations where objects rotate, rotary stability is proportional to angular momentum. Rotary stability increases as mass and angular velocity increase, and as mass is extended farther from the axis of rotation.

REVIEW QUESTIONS

1. Stand with your back, seat, and heels against a wall. Keep your legs extended and bend down to touch your toes. Why do you topple forward? Explain what occurs in terms of the line of your center of gravity and your base of support. Step clear of the wall and perform the same action; explain why you can now maintain your balance.

2. Why is rotary stability a battle of one torque versus another? As an example in your answer, use an athlete balancing on one foot on the beam.

3. Using the example of a defending wrestler lying on a wrestling mat, explain why stability increases when he extends his base of support in the direction of force (and torque) applied by an attacker.

4. Skills that require an athlete to change direction suddenly or be ready to thrust in any direction require the athlete to assume a position that does not have maximal stability. Why is this true?

5. When a discus is rotating, its stability depends on its angular momentum. Why?

6. An Olympic weight lifter weighing 200 lb stands erect with his feet together and with a 400 lb barbell at arm's length above his head. Why is it difficult for the weight lifter in this situation to maintain a state of equilibrium and control the barbell?

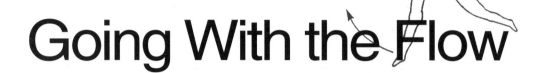

CHAPTER 6

Going With the Flow

When you finish reading this chapter, you should be able to explain

- how the fluid forces of hydrostatic pressure, buoyancy, drag, and lift affect athletes and objects as they move through air and water;

- how pressure, temperature, and the nature of air and water affect the way fluids act;

- how surface drag, form drag, and wave drag affect the movements of athletes and objects through air and water;

- how competitors in high velocity sports counteract or make use of drag and lift; and

- how the magnus effect and drag forces affect the flight path of a spinning ball.

We could just as well call this chapter "Going Against the Flow" because it deals with the way the forces of air and water can help or hinder an athlete. In the following pages you'll read about swimmers using the resistance of water to maximize their propulsion, and you'll learn why one athlete can be a floater and another a sinker. You'll learn why competitive cyclists use aerobars, disc wheels, and slick racing suits and why discus throwers love to compete in stadia where they can launch the discus into a head wind. You'll also read how a pitcher uses spin to produce a curveball and why golf balls travel farther and faster when they're covered in dimples rather than being smooth. This chapter is about making the most of the flow!

Hundreds of sports take a real interest in the forces produced by air and water. They range from the underwater sport of scuba diving to speed events like downhill skiing, and from high-speed events like auto racing and cycling to high-flying sports like hot air ballooning and parachute jumping.

In contrast, you'll find many sports in which the forces exerted by air and water play little part in the outcome of the competition. Wrestlers don't worry about air resistance when they're pinning an opponent, and gymnasts don't move along a beam at speeds that require them to be streamlined! The same can be said about basketball. Basketball players would have to play on an outdoor court in a gale before they'd worry about the effect of wind on the quality of their performance.

Although air is obviously not as thick and dense as water, both act like fluids. They flow around and easily mold to the shape of an athlete or an object. Allowing for differences in intensity, this characteristic means that air and water exert similar forces. These forces are hydrostatic pressure, buoyancy, drag, and lift. Let's look at each of these and see how they affect athletic performance.

Hydrostatic Pressure

Hydrostatic pressure is the force exerted by a fluid, like air or water. To understand hydrostatic pressure, let's look at our own atmosphere. Most of us don't think of the atmosphere around us as weighing down on our bodies, but it does! The easiest way to imagine this concept is to think of the atmosphere like blankets layered on you when you're lying in bed. Each blanket rests on top of another and each blanket holds up those above and presses down on those below. Imagine your bed as the surface of the earth with you resting on the bed. At sea level you have the most blankets of atmosphere on top of you. At high altitudes, you have one or two blankets lying on you instead of several. If you go up high enough, it's like throwing off all the blankets of atmosphere! In other words, the greatest atmospheric pressure exists at sea level and it gets less as you go up. At sea level, the weight of the atmosphere is approximately 14.7 lb on every square inch of the earth's surface. In the metric system, 14.7 lb per square inch is just over 100 KPa (kilopascals). 14.7 psi (lb per square inch) presses on every square inch of you too! So if you'd measured the area of the top of your head (and forgot the rest of your body!), you could work out the weight of the atmosphere pressing down just on your head. For adults this can be more than 1,000 lb! As hu-

mans we've evolved so that we can put up with this kind of pressure. You don't feel it, but you'd be in big trouble if this pressure was ever removed!

When you start going to high altitudes, take your time and allow yourself to become acclimatized to air that has lower pressure and gives you less oxygen with each breath. Tourists who casually decide to climb Mt. Kilimanjaro as part of a trip to Kenya will attest to this! We've already talked about the benefits and detrimental effects of altitude for athletes in chapter 2.

Water is much more dense than air and a cubic foot of salt water will weigh more than a cubic foot of fresh water. Because water weighs so much more than an equivalent amount of air, the pressure exerted by water increases with depth much faster than in air. Scuba divers learn that for every 33 ft they go down in the ocean, the pressure increases the equivalent of one atmosphere (i.e., 14.7 psi). So at 33 ft you have the 14.7 lb that exists at the surface of the ocean added to another 14.7 lb for a total of 29.4 psi. At 66 ft the pressure increases to 44.1 psi, and at 99 ft it's squeezing the diver with a pressure of 58.8 lb on every square inch of the diver's body (see Figure 6.1). The greater part of the diver's body can put up with this pressure, but not so the diver's air cavities. The sinuses, lungs, and inner ear all have air cavities, and pressure in these areas must be balanced with whatever pressure the water exerts. A healthy diver (who doesn't have a cold blocking a sinus), who descends slowly, breathing regularly through a scuba regulator, has no problem equalizing the pressure in the body with what's outside.

When scuba divers descend deep in the ocean, the air they breathe must be at the same pressure as the pressure of the surrounding water. As all scuba divers should know, breathing air at high pressure produces conditions that can be potentially dangerous. Air is almost 79% nitrogen and with the high pressures experienced at depth a considerable amount gets dissolved into the bloodstream. If the diver stays at depth for long, there is a possibility of suffering "raptures of the deep" or "nitrogen narcosis." This is a condition in which nitrogen acts like having too much alcohol. It affects the nervous system making the diver disoriented and irrational.

Problems also exist for a scuba diver on the way up. If the diver rises too rapidly, nitrogen

Atmospheric pressure = 14.7 lb per square inch (psi)

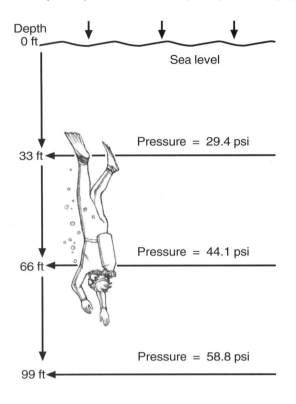

Fig. 6.1. Pressure increases by one atmosphere (14.7 psi) for every 33 ft of depth.

bubbles may not be expired properly through the lungs. Instead they lodge in the spine, joints, and muscles. This produces a condition descriptively and painfully known as the "bends" because the diver can be crippled and bent over. A diver avoids this condition by having enough air in reserve to ascend slowly and make decompression stops to allow the nitrogen to be safely discharged. A gradual reduction in pressure allows nitrogen to be transported to the lungs for elimination.

We need to mention one other important characteristic of scuba diving. One lungful of air at 33 ft expands to twice its size at the surface. At 66 ft one lungful of air becomes 3 lungsful at the surface, and at 99 ft a single lungful expands to 4 times its size at the surface! So a scuba diver who sucks his tank dry at 99 ft, then holds his breath to the surface, can expect the air in his lungs to expand 4 times its size by the time he gets to the surface. There's no way the lungs can handle this expansion! Scuba divers avoid this very dangerous situation by breathing normally

on the way up and always having sufficient air in the tank to avoid rush ascents.

Buoyancy

Buoyancy is related to hydrostatic pressure, and it is one of the few forces that lifts upward and fights gravity. When an athlete or an object is fully immersed in water, the water presses on the athlete from all directions. Because pressure in a fluid increases with depth, there's more pressure pushing on the athlete from below than there is from the sides, or from above. The result is that there is a more powerful upward force pushing on the athlete from below. This is the force of **buoyancy**.

Keep in mind that buoyancy doesn't only apply to water. Buoyancy exists in the air too. Hot air ballooning is a sport that is based on the fact that a volume of hot air weighs less than an equivalent amount of surrounding cooler air. When you sit in the stadium seats and watch a television blimp circling overhead, you are looking at an object filled with a gas (helium), which is lighter than air. The blimp rises in the air because a buoyant force is acting on it.

Because numerous sports like swimming, rowing, kayaking, and yachting are affected by the buoyant force of water, let's look at how it works. There's a simple principle that will tell you how strong the upward lift of buoyancy is going to be. The buoyant force acting on an athlete immersed in water is equal to the weight of the water that the athlete's body takes the place of, or pushes out of the way. If the athlete displaces a lot of water, the buoyant force pushing upward is increased. When the buoyant force is greater than the force of gravity pulling the athlete down, the athlete is pushed to the surface (see Figure 6.2). This means that an athlete will float if the athlete weighs 200 lb and the water the athlete displaces weighs more than 200 lb. This principle becomes really interesting when you watch what happens to athletes of different body types floating in the pool. An athlete who has big bones, big muscles, and very little fat has a lot of mass squashed into the space that the athlete's body occupies. A cubic inch of bone and muscle is more dense and weighs more than the same amount of fat. An athlete with a body type that is predominately bone and muscle is likely to weigh more than the water the athlete displaces. Consequently, gravity pulls down more than the buoyant force pushes up and the athlete sinks! You used to see these types of athletes featured on television in superstar competitions. Huge, muscular athletes, who are best at land sports, turn the swimming competition into a submarine race because most of them are sinkers! The buoyant force acting on their bodies loses to gravity. But if these superstars left the pool and competed in the ocean, there'd be a good chance they'd be floaters. Because of its additional salt content, the water the athletes displace in the ocean weighs more than the fresh water they displaced in the pool. If the amount of the displaced ocean water weighs more than they do, then they'll float.

The percent body fat that an athlete possesses plays an important role in distance swimming, particularly in colder ocean waters. It not only helps to keep them at the surface, but it also keeps them warm. Vicki Keith, the phenomenal Canadian distance swimmer who swam all the frigid Great Lakes in Canada (using the butterfly all the way!), had a high percent body fat. Body fat not only assists in buoyancy but, coupled with a coating of grease the athlete spreads over her body, resists the loss of body heat and the onset of hypothermia. An athlete with minimal body fat suffers from hypothermia more quickly than an athlete who has a high proportion of body fat.

If you give a wet suit to an athlete who has a low percent body fat, you'd find that the athlete has an easier time staying afloat. A wet suit increases the athlete's space in the water with little increase in weight because the wet suit weighs very little. The thicker the wet suit the greater the space (or **volume**) the athlete takes up. So the buoyant force pushing up is increased with little change in the athlete's body weight.

If an athlete wearing a wet suit descends well below the surface of the ocean, the increased pressure with depth compresses the suit. The deeper the athlete goes, the more compression. In this situation the athlete can become a sinker. Scuba divers wear lead hip weights to counter the additional buoyancy of the wet suit when they're at the surface. As they descend, the increased pressure compresses the wet suit. Scuba divers balance the loss of buoyancy that occurs by pumping air from their tanks into what is called "a buoyancy vest." The expanded buoyancy vest increases the space they take up in the water and so the buoyant force is increased as well. Too much air in the buoyancy vest and the scuba diver rises to the surface. On the other hand, if the diver wants to hang in the water like an astronaut in space, she pumps just enough air into the vest to balance the upward push of the buoyant force against the downward pull of gravity.

All of us can use our lungs as a mini buoyancy vest. If an athlete takes a really deep breath and expands the rib cage, she takes up more space in the water. The buoyant force is increased without any change in body weight. For many athletes (but not all) this action is sufficient to hold them at the surface. Exhaling reverses the situation and the athlete starts to sink. This phenomenon can be tested quite easily in a swimming pool.

The buoyant force acting on an athlete varies according to fluid thickness (i.e., density), and according to fluid temperature. The warmer the fluid, the less dense it becomes. So it's easier to float in a cold salty ocean than in warm fresh water. Cold ocean water is more

Weight of swimmer

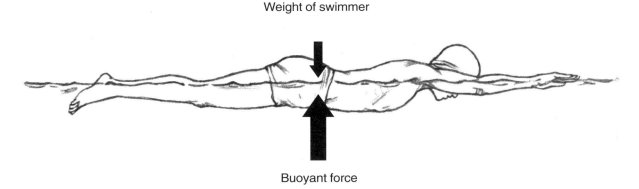

Buoyant force

Fig. 6.2.   When the buoyant force is greater than gravity's downward pull (i.e., the athlete's weight), the athlete will float.

Breath-hold Diving

The world record for descending below the surface of the ocean on a single breath of air is now in excess of 400 ft. Divers in this sport hyperventilate on the surface and then hurtle downward into the cold and darkness, clinging to a heavy weight that slides on a cable hooked to the ocean floor. They then climb hand over hand up the cable or inflate an air bag that drags them back to the surface. On the way down they are forced to equalize the intense pressure, which at 400 ft presses on their eardrums at close to 200 psi. The present record holder, Francisco Ferreras, is able to breath-hold for 7 min and to conserve oxygen as his heart rate slows from 60 beats/min at the surface to 3 to 4 beats/min at 400 ft. Ferreras feels he can pass 500 ft. By comparison, sperm whales, the world's deepest diving mammals, have been recorded at depths in excess of 7,000 ft.

---

dense and weighs more than an equal volume of fresh water. In cold ocean water there is a greater likelihood that the amount of water displaced by an athlete will weigh more than the athlete does!

Center of Buoyancy

The place where the buoyant force concentrates its upward push on an athlete's body is called the **center of buoyancy**. An athlete's torso and upper body contain the lungs and collectively take up plenty of space in the water. In comparison to an athlete's legs, the upper body takes up more space and weighs less than the water it displaces. Consequently, the upper body is pushed upward more than the athlete's legs. The result is that the center of buoyancy for most athletes is not the same place as the center of gravity, but higher, generally just below the rib cage.

Floating Position

The position an athlete assumes when floating is determined by the fact that the center of buoyancy is higher on the body than the athlete's center of gravity. Normally the buoyant force concentrates its upward push just below the rib cage while gravity pulls downward at approximately waist level. These two forces, one acting up and the other down, cause rotation. The athlete's legs drop downward while the chest lifts up. Rotation ceases when the two forces are aligned with the center of buoyancy directly above the center of gravity. The chest is up and the lower body and legs hang beneath. Figure 6.3a shows gravity pulling down and buoyancy pushing up on a swimmer. The alignment of the pull of gravity and the buoyant force acting on the swimmer is shown in Figure 6.3b.

The tendency of an athlete's body to rotate is magnified when an athlete's legs are muscular and lean. A swimmer who has muscular legs with little fat must counter the legs' desire to sink with an efficient leg kick to maintain a streamlined body position. Without a good kick the legs drop, which increases drag from the water. Figure 6.4a shows an inefficient swimming position in which the athlete's body is angled downward with the legs low in the water. When the athlete's body is parallel to the direction of movement, the resistance from the water is dramatically reduced (see Figure 6.4b).

Lean muscular athletes such as you see in triathlon competitions find that negative buoyancy is not much of a problem in the ocean. In many triathlons athletes are allowed to use thin "farmer-john" style wet suits that give freedom to their arms for swimming but still act like a coating of body fat. These wet suits not only keep the athlete warm but also improve buoyancy. The increased buoyancy in salt water coupled with the help from the wet suit pushes the athlete's body (particularly their legs) into a streamlined position. As a result their swimming stroke is more efficient and they consume less energy.

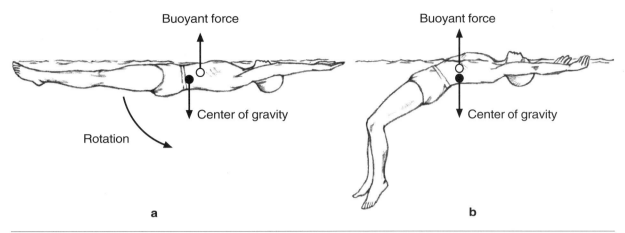

Fig. 6.3. Torque caused by the forces of gravity and buoyancy makes an athlete rotate to a floating position where the center of buoyancy is directly above the center of gravity.
Reprinted from Luttgens et al. 1992.

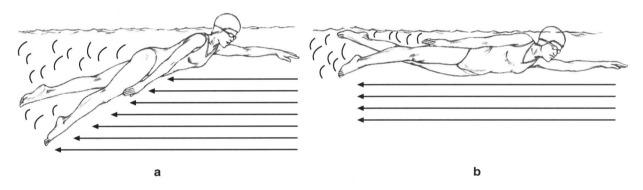

Fig. 6.4. In swimming, considerable drag is caused by a low leg position (a). A high leg position (b) reduces drag.

World records swum in salt water pools have been disallowed because the buoyancy of salt water is such a help to the athlete. Even though ocean water is more dense (around 2.5%) and offers more resistance than fresh water, the streamlined body position of an elite swimmer lying flat and high in salt water produces faster times than in fresh water. Swim officials are well aware of this. There are even rules specifying the amount of salt allowed in a fresh water swimming pool!

Drag

In most cases **drag** is a "drag" because it's a collection of fluid forces that tend to oppose the actions an athlete is trying to perform. Drag pushes, pulls, and tugs on an athlete. If an athlete runs to

the left, drag forces act to the right. Whatever the direction, drag forces act in opposition. It's easy to guess what will increase these drag forces. If an athlete like Olympic champion Gail Devers sprints faster, the air is going to push and pull at her more. If she sprints along the beach and then runs into the water as occurs at the start of triathlons, the drag on her body is greater in the water than in the air.

Drag varies according to the type of fluid (water or air), and whether the fluid is warm or cold, and how dense and viscous, (sticky and clinging) it is. Drag also depends on the size and shape of the athlete. A giant sprinter wearing a full-length fur coat that grabs at the wind is going to generate more drag than a smaller athlete in a slick, polished bodysuit.

Let's look at each aspect of drag. We'll start by examining the velocity of the athlete and the fluid. When you consider drag, it's important to remember that it doesn't matter what or who's doing the moving—it can be the athlete or the fluid, or both. If the fluid is moving, then drag occurs even when an athlete is standing still! As you'll see, what's important is the relative motion that takes place between the fluid and the athlete.

Relative Motion

Elite swimmers practice in special tanks called "flumes." A turbine drives the water past their bodies. The swimmers swim hard but go nowhere—the water does the moving! In a swimming pool the reverse occurs. The water is stationary. The swimmers travel through and past the water. In a flowing river you can have a situation where the water moves and so do the swimmers! These three situations (swimming in the flume, the pool, and the river), give you the following variations in what is called **relative motion**.

1. In the flume, the water moves past the swimmers. The swimmers stay in the same spot. The water moves.
2. In the pool, the swimmers move past the water. The water is stationary. The swimmers move.
3. In the river, swimmers and water move.

Relative motion is the motion of one item relative to another, and in our examples, one item is a swimmer and the other is the water. In these situations, if the relative movement of swimmer and water past each other is the same, then the drag forces produced are the same also. In other words, drag forces can be the same no matter who or what's doing the moving!

Let's look at this concept of relative motion a little further. Figure 6.5 shows three variations in relative motion. In 6.5a an athlete is sprinting at 20 mph into a head wind of 5 mph. You can see that the athlete moves one direction at 20 mph and airflow is in the opposite direction at 5 mph. The relative velocity of airflow past the athlete in this situation is 25 mph. In Figure 6.5b the athlete sprints at 20 mph but with a following wind of 5 mph. The relative velocity of airflow past the athlete is now 15 mph. In Figure 6.5c the athlete is again sprinting at 20 mph but with a following wind of 20 mph. The relative velocity of the airflow past the athlete in this situation is zero. Why? Because both athlete and airflow are traveling in

the same direction at the same velocity. In the three examples we've just described, the greatest frictional forces acting on the athlete occur in Figure 6.5a and minimally in Figure 6.5c.

The fact that similar force characteristics can occur whether the athlete moves or the fluid moves is the principle employed not only in flumes but also in wind tunnels. Wind tunnels are used to assess drag forces that occur when athletes (plus their equipment), move at high speed through the air. Just as a coach checks a swimmer's technique by watching through an observation window in the flume, so wind tunnels can be used to perfect the aerodynamic qualities of athletes like Tour de France winner Greg LeMond and world speed skating champion Bonnie Blair. When air is driven past Greg and Bonnie in the wind tunnel, it gives an assessment of the drag forces that occur when Greg and Bonnie are doing the moving!

Wind tunnels give valuable data on how to reduce the drag produced by fluid forces. They also provide information on whether fluid forces (like drag and lift) can be used in some way. This information is then used in such sports as auto racing, gliding, ski jumping, and in throwing events like the javelin and discus. It is common knowledge to throwers and to track and field coaches that a discus travels farther when it is spun at release and launched (like a glider) at an appropriate angle into a head wind. Wind tunnel tests can determine the discus's optimal trajectory and its flight position and spin relative to wind velocity and wind direction. With each change in wind velocity and direction, so the angle of release and flight characteristics of the discus have to change. From wind tunnel tests using a stationary spinning discus, and from practical experimentation by throwers, it has been found that a head wind of about 15 to 20 mph can add 20 ft or more to the distance thrown, compared with throwing in still air. Consequently, athletes try to adjust the flight of the discus according to the conditions that they meet. Astute discus throwers quickly learn which venues have winds that blow regularly from a favorable direction. They then try to compete at that venue as often as possible.

Characteristics of Air and Water

Both air and water vary in consistency. Air is obviously not as thick, dense, or sticky as water, but

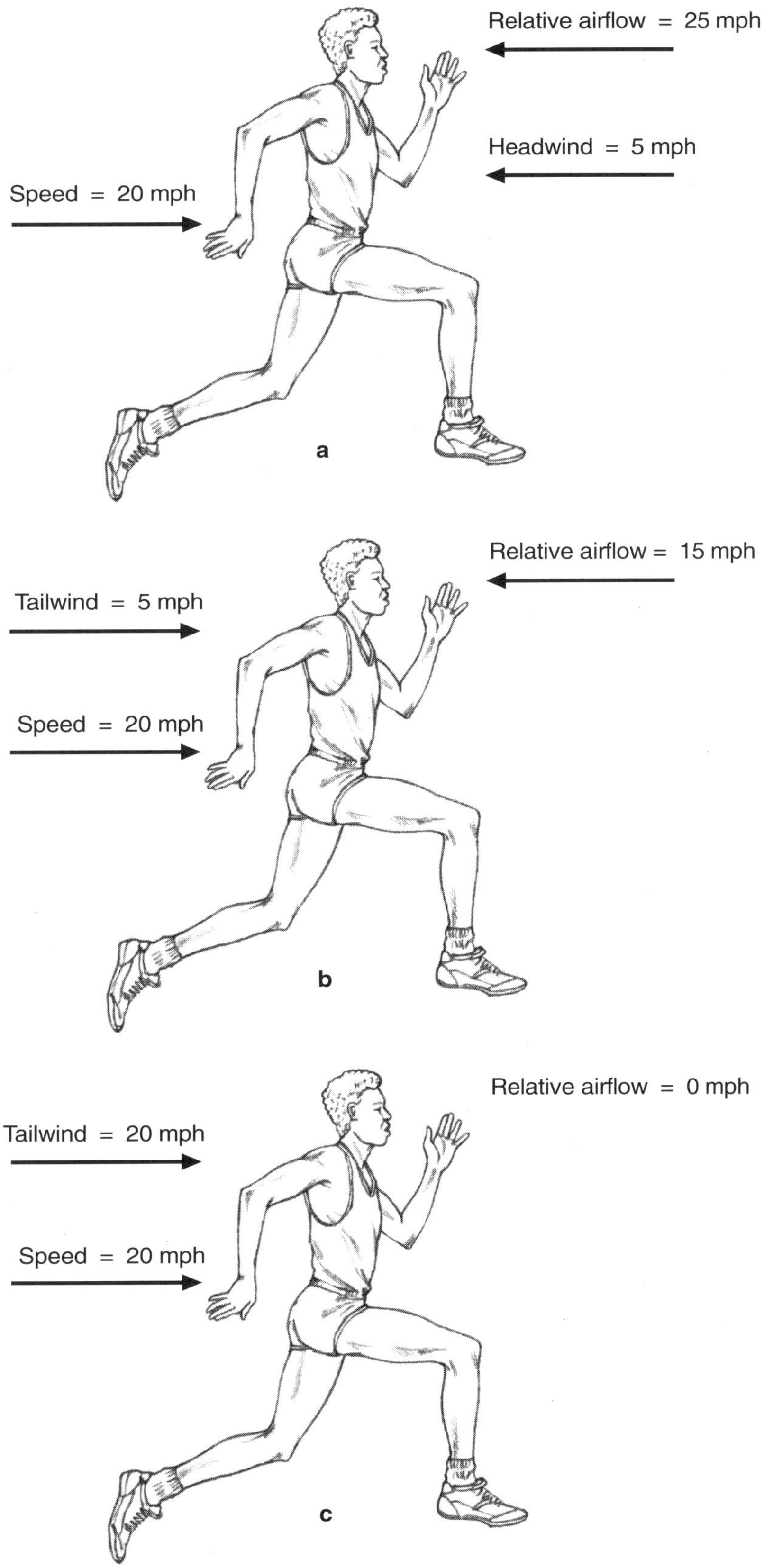

Fig. 6.5.   Three examples of relative motion in sprinting.

both air and water vary in density. Pressure variations, temperature changes, and differences in what air and water contain (like water droplets in the air and salt in water), all change the way these fluids act and the way they affect sport performances.

Athletes compete when it's hot or cold, from sea level to high altitude, and at times when humidity (i.e., the percentage of water vapor in the air) is high. Variations in these conditions affect how fast athletes move, how far baseballs fly, and how much movement can be put on a curveball or a knuckleball. Because there are so many variations of pressure, temperature, and humidity, let's look at a summary of what happens.

When air temperature rises, the air thins out and its density decreases. When this happens the resistance air puts up against a moving object decreases. If barometric pressure (i.e., air pressure) increases, then its density increases and its resistance against a moving object increases too. We've already discussed that air pressure is normally greatest at sea level. It gets less as you move to higher altitudes. So you experience less resistance from the air the higher you go. When humidity increases, the density of the air *decreases*. This may seem contrary to what you'd think, yet it's true. Brancazio (1984) writes, "You may find this surprising, since the air often feels 'heavy' on humid days—but this feeling arises from body physiology (perspiration evaporates more slowly when the air is damp) and not from the actual density of the air. In damp air, oxygen and nitrogen molecules are replaced by lighter-weight water molecules." So humid air is less dense and moving objects are subject to less resistance than in dry air of the same temperature and pressure. Of course everything changes when humidity switches to precipitation. In a heavy downpour, water is no longer in a vapor state and a baseball has to push its way through the rain. In this situation the ball has to contend with the additional resistance of falling rain.

What these atmospheric characteristics tell us is that an athlete or an object like a baseball or a golf ball will travel faster and farther in warm conditions than cold, faster and farther at high altitude than at sea level, and faster and farther on a humid day than a dry day. It's for this reason that batters hit farther and pitchers fire in fastballs faster in Denver, where the ballpark is well above sea level. On the other hand, pitchers hurling curveballs and knuckleballs need thick air that grabs at the seams of the ball and helps to move the ball around. What's good for a fastball doesn't produce the fluttering deception of a knuckleball! You'll see why later in this chapter.

Just as a fastball will go faster at high altitude, so will a sprint cyclist. Allowing for the lack of oxygen at high altitude, most cycling records from 200 m sprint to the 1 hr time trial were set at high altitude in places like Colorado Springs or Mexico City. Now cycling records set at high altitude are considered second class and not as good as those set at sea level. To receive the full accolades of the cycling fraternity, it's better to set them at close to sea level as Miguel Indurain did in Bordeaux, France. Miguel, a multiple winner of the Tour de France, flashed around the Bordeaux track to break the 1 hr cycling record. The distance he covered in an hour was 53.04 km. This means that Miguel averaged 32.95 miles an hour!

The consistency of water differs just as it does for air. Water varies in density depending on the proportions of other substances it contains. An athlete attempting to swim in the Dead Sea in Jordan will be shocked at the difference between the water there and the water in a swimming pool. The Dead Sea is incredibly thick and dense because of its high salt content. Even the leanest and most muscular athlete can lie back in the water, and with little to no movement, read the *Mechanics of Sport* without fear of sinking!

Fluid Viscosity

Viscosity is a measure of a fluid's flow. You can think of viscosity as a fluid's stickiness and its ability to cling to the surface of an object. Air is obviously less sticky than water but air differs from water in that its viscosity increases slightly with an increase in temperature whereas the viscosity of water is reduced with an increase in temperature. The viscosity of water and air plays a big part in what is called surface drag. Surface drag combines with two other types of drag, called form drag and wave drag, to make up the three most important drag forces that affect the movement of an athlete or an object. Let's look at each of these types of drag.

Surface Drag

Surface drag is also called viscous drag, or skin friction. These names immediately tell you how surface drag works. When an athlete or an object moves through a fluid, the fluid forms what is called a **boundary layer**, which because of the fluid's viscosity, drags and clings to the surface of whatever it contacts. Figure 6.6 shows the boundary layer around a ball that is moving slowly through the air.

If an athlete moves through air or water, the athlete drags and pushes at the fluid, and the fluid does the same thing to the athlete. In cycling, the air that comes into direct contact with champions Greg LeMond or Rebecca Twigg as they cycle is slowed because Greg, Rebecca, and their bicycles exert a force on the air. The air exerts an equal and opposite force on them. It's this return force, called a "reaction force," that constitutes surface drag. A similar situation occurs when Janet Evans and Pablo Morales swim in the pool.

The boundary layer of fluid that is slowed by an athlete then slows its adjacent layer. This process continues outward until the effect is finally dissipated.

The amount of surface drag developed by an athlete's movements depends on how viscous or sticky the fluid is, how big a surface area the athlete exposes to the flow, how rough the athlete's surfaces are, and the relative velocity of the athlete and the fluid. So the stickier the fluid, the bigger and rougher the athlete's surfaces are, and the faster both athlete and fluid move past each other, the greater the surface drag.

Form Drag

To surface drag we now add its close associate—**form drag**. Form drag is also called shape drag,

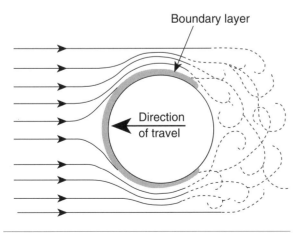

Fig. 6.6. Boundary layer around a ball traveling through the air.

profile drag, and pressure drag. As these names suggest, form drag is produced by the shape and size of an athlete and his equipment like Greg LeMond pedaling his bicycle as he pushes through the air, or Janet Evans as she propels herself through water. If Greg and Janet travel fast enough, their bodies, pushing through the air and water, cause an area of turbulence to occur behind them. This area, called the **wake** (like the wake to the rear of a ship), is a region of swirling low pressure and suction. If you've ever been cycling on a highway, you'll have experienced this swirling low pressure when a big 18 wheeler passed by!

Ahead of Greg and Janet as they move along is an area of high pressure. This occurs where they hit the air and water head-on. The amount of form drag they experience depends on the difference between the high pressure in front of them and the low pressure behind. More high pressure and more low pressure means more form drag.

It's easy to guess what increases an athlete's form drag. Form drag increases the faster an athlete and fluid flow past each other. It also increases according to how thick, dense, and sticky the fluid is. If the athlete maintains a shape that increases the high pressure in front and the low pressure to the rear, then this too will increase form drag. What kind of shape are we talking about here? Think of Greg LeMond pedaling as fast as possible into a strong wind sitting bolt upright on an old-fashioned bicycle. His upright body and high velocity would cause a large high pressure area to develop in front of him and a huge turbulent low pressure area to the rear. Greg's form drag on the old bicycle would be enormous. If he wore loose, flapping clothing and strapped huge carrier bags and luggage to his bike, his surface drag would be enormous too. It wouldn't be long before he ran out of energy trying to battle the combined effect of these drag forces.

Efforts to reduce surface and form drag occur in sport wherever large shapes and surfaces move at high speed. That's why in so many sports you see body positions and equipment that are designed to

- eliminate pushing through air or water with a blunt shape having a large cross-sectional area;
- eliminate lumps, bumps, projections, and rough edges;
- smooth out surfaces; and
- fill in the area at the rear of the athlete or object where the low pressure wake occurs.

It's for these reasons that designers aim for a streamlined teardrop or egg shape with smooth surfaces in events like cycling, skiing, auto racing, luge, and boat racing. Figure 6.7, a and b, compares the flow patterns around the blunt circular shape of a ball and a teardrop shape. Notice in Figure 6.7a that a ball shape produces a turbulent wake area at its rear and in Figure 6.7b that the teardrop shape causes the flow patterns to fill in and eliminate this turbulent area.

Let's look closely at the sport of cycling to see how these design features work. Elite athletes like multiple Tour de France winner Miguel Indurain ride bikes made of lightweight metals and modern composite materials. The bike frame is often raked (i.e., tilted downward toward the front wheel) and equipped with a larger rear wheel and extended handlebars. The combination of these features forces the rider into a sleek aerodynamic position with the back parallel to the ground. The athlete's head is lowered and the arms extended. This flattened cycling position lessens high pressure in front and makes the cyclist simulate a dart in order to cut through the air with the hands and arms leading the way.

To reduce surface friction, the athlete wears a low-friction, single piece skintight suit with no wrinkles or loose flapping sections. Skintight fingerless gloves and laceless shoes, or booties, are also worn. Legs, arms, and face are shaved. A teardrop aerodynamic helmet is worn. Sometimes the helmet is blade shaped to slice through the air. Disc coverings are used on the rear wheel. The front wheel is made of lightweight composite material and has only three large spokes each with a teardrop cross section. This design is intended to reduce the immense egg-beater drag caused by regular spoke patterns. All other components on the bike are in aerodynamic teardrop shapes and, wherever possible, items like cables are totally hidden in the frame. For those cyclists looking for the ultimate in assistance, their bodies are sprayed with silicone!

Downhill speed skiers, who attempt to reach the greatest possible velocity over a measured course, are similar to cyclists in their efforts to minimize drag forces. Their crouched body positions, body-contoured poles with minimal size baskets, superslick uniforms, and aerodynamic helmets and boots are all designed to reduce form and surface drag.

Even with all these modifications to beat drag, cyclists using equipment and body positions similar to those described above are not as aerodynamically efficient as those who cycle in a recumbent (i.e., inclined or lying) position and cover themselves totally with lightweight shells or fairings. Using these human-powered vehicles, athletes can pedal more than 65 mph, far faster than the world's best sprint cyclist. To date, lightweight shells and fairings are not allowed in the Tour de France or in Olympic cycling competitions. For the average person, cycling in a recumbent position inside a lightweight shell would make cycling faster and less energy consuming. But being lower down, they're difficult for motorists to see, and they get blown around in crosswinds!

When you stand in front of one of these human-powered vehicles, you notice how narrow they are. This narrow, pointed profile reduces the cross-sectional area at the front of the vehicle and the high pressure that occurs there. The sides of the shells and fairings are smooth, polished, and slick, and all vehicles are designed to have a long, tapering tail. The tapering tail fills in the low pressure wake that occurs to the rear of the vehicle. The objective is the same as the skier, to reduce form and surface drag to a minimum (see Figure 6.8).

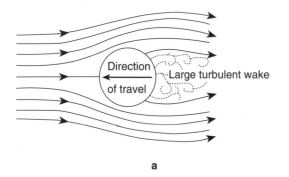

a

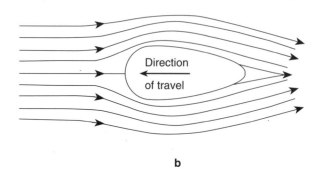

b

Fig. 6.7.   A teardrop shape eliminates the turbulent low pressure wake that occurs to the rear of a circular shape (like a ball).

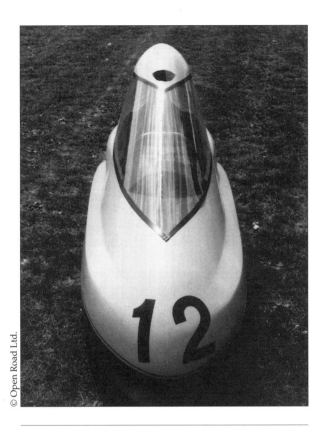

Fig. 6.8. High speed human-powered vehicle.

Similar to the human-powered vehicles, luge competitors lying back on their small toboggans even worry about their noses sticking up and the drag caused by the shape of their faces. Even though an athlete's nose is small compared with the rest of the athlete's body, it's still a projection and increases drag. To counter this problem, athletes cover their faces with plastic shields. It's

worth the effort, particularly when .01 sec frequently separates one medal from the next.

Making use of the wake. In cycle pursuit races, two teams start on opposing sides of the track and attempt to gain distance on each other. In each team the leading cyclist expends more energy carving through the air than do the remaining members on the team. The second cyclist drafts in the low pressure wake of the first cyclist. The third cyclist does the same behind the second and likewise the fourth behind the third. As the team races around the oval, the leading cyclist drops to the rear and the second in line takes up the task of leading. In this way each team member conserves energy by drafting behind their teammates.

The benefit of drafting is that the drafting athlete can keep up the same speed as the lead cyclist, while expending less energy. In essence the drafting cyclist has very little high pressure in front and is pulled along in the wake that trails the cyclist in front. This technique is often called "slipstreaming."

The closer the drafting cyclist follows the lead cyclist, the better. Distances less than 12 in between the rear tire of the lead cyclist and the front wheel of the drafting athlete are most efficient. One reason that a tandem is faster than a single cyclist is that the rear rider on a tandem is drafting behind his partner. Even though there is a greater surface area exposed to the air in a tandem, the additional power of two riders and the benefits of drafting produce faster speeds than single cyclists.

In triathlon competitions, the benefits experienced by the drafting athlete are so enormous that drafting is forbidden during the cycling part of

Drafting Takes Cyclist John Howard to 152 mph!

No factor demonstrates the advantages of drafting more clearly than the top speeds attained by cyclists with and without drafting. The best time for 200 m from a flying start is 9.86 sec by Curt Harnett of Canada. Harnett's speed of just over 45 mph was managed without drafting behind a pace vehicle. Compare Harnett's efforts with the incredible 152.28 mph John Howard of the United States attained when he drafted behind a specially designed race car on the Bonneville Salt Flats in 1985! Howard needed no streamlining because he was pulled along in the suction to the rear of the pace vehicle. He also used a unique double chainwheel arrangement on his bicycle so that he could pedal at 152 mph!

the race. Similar regulations exist in the Tour de France. Although cyclists are allowed to draft behind each other, they are not allowed to get assistance from motorized vehicles. In the 1993 Women's Tour de France, Jeannie Longo of France, at that time the world's greatest female cyclist, was penalized for drafting behind a motorcycle!

How drag affects the flight of baseballs, tennis balls, and golf balls. If you examine what happens to a smooth-surfaced ball as it travels through the air and what happens to a ball with seams (like a baseball), or dimples (like a golf ball), you find that some dramatic differences occur in the way that drag affects each ball. These changes play an important role in determining the flight of baseballs, tennis balls, and golf balls.

You'll notice that a circular and blunt object like a ball is poorly streamlined and produces considerable drag. In addition, you can't change a ball's shape in the way that you can redesign a racing car or a bobsled so they become more aerodynamic. A ball is always ball shaped no matter how small or how large.

To understand what happens, let's have a smooth-surfaced ball move through the air very slowly. At this velocity the boundary layer of air that contacts the surface of the ball flows smoothly around the ball. Its flow pattern looks like laminations in a piece of plywood. This type of flow pattern is called **laminar** or streamlined. Moving at such a low velocity, the drag affecting the ball is predominately surface drag caused by the clinging nature of the boundary layer (see Figure 6.9).

If we make the ball travel faster so the velocity of airflow around the ball increases, the laminar flow starts to break up. Smooth laminar flow is now mixed with a disturbed, distorted, **turbulent flow** pattern. Because of the higher velocity

with which air passes the ball, the air cannot follow the ball's contours the same way it did when it passed slowly. Instead, the boundary layer follows the ball's contours part way; thereafter it tears away from the ball's surface toward the rear of the ball. This causes a turbulent low pressure wake to develop at the rear. With the increase in velocity that air and ball pass each other, pressure also builds up where the ball hits the air head-on. So we have high pressure increasing at the front and low pressure increasing at the rear. The net result is that the ball experiences more form drag (see Figure 6.10).

If the ball and the air travel by each other at an even greater velocity, the place where the boundary layer breaks away from the ball's surface moves *from the rear of the ball toward the front*. The result is an even bigger wake area at the rear. There's more high pressure at the front of the ball and more low pressure at the rear, so form drag increases significantly (see Figure 6.11).

Finally, if the ball and air pass each other at really high velocity, the boundary layer becomes totally turbulent. Now a surprising change happens! When the boundary layer is totally turbulent, the place where it separates from the ball shifts *back toward the rear* and reduces the size of the low pressure wake. The result is that the ball's form drag reduces also (see Figure 6.12).

This characteristic is important to games like tennis, baseball, and golf because a ball covered with fuzz, seams, or dimples causes a turbulent

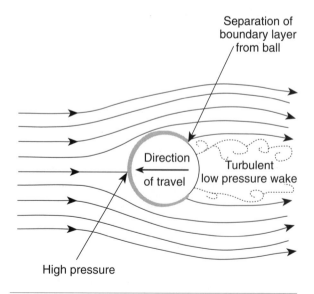

Fig. 6.10. Turbulent flow pattern. At *high* velocities the boundary layer breaks away to the rear of the ball, causing a low pressure wake.

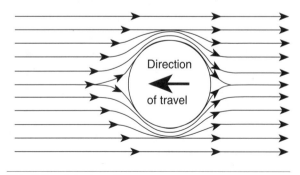

Fig. 6.9. Laminar flow.

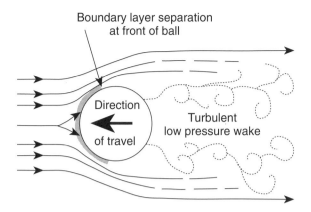

Fig. 6.11. Turbulent flow pattern. At *higher* velocities the boundary layer shifts to the front of the ball.

boundary layer to form all around the ball—not only at high velocities but at low velocities as well. So fuzz, seams, and dimples reduce form drag and help the ball fly farther and faster and hold to its flight path better than if the ball were smooth all over. It's true that roughing up the surface of the ball in this manner causes surface drag to increase, but the total drag affecting the ball is less because of the reduction in form drag (see Figure 6.12). When spin is put on the ball, which is a big part of tennis, baseball and golf, the ball curves better in flight and holds to the curve better than if the ball were smooth. When we look at how a pitcher throws curveballs you'll see how this occurs.

Wave Drag

The third and final type of drag acts at the interface where water and air meet. It is called **wave**

drag and affects swimming (particularly breaststroke and butterfly where there can be a lot of up and down motion) and other water sports like rowing, kayaking, and yachting. When a swimmer moves through the water, waves in front of the swimmer create a high pressure wall of water that resists the swimmer's forward motion. The larger the cross-sectional area that the swimmer pushes into the water, the larger is the wall of water opposing the swimmer. So if the swimmer acts like a barge bashing its way through the water, the wave drag will be phenomenal!

At competitive speeds, wave drag is far worse than surface and form drag. Surface and form drag increase according to the *square* of the velocity. This means, for example, that if a swimmer doubles her velocity through the water, surface and form drag increase fourfold. Wave drag, on the other hand, increases according to the *cube* of the velocity. So, if a swimmer doubles her velocity, wave drag increases eight-fold (i.e. $2 \times 2 \times 2$). If the swimmer were to triple her velocity, wave drag would increase $3 \times 3 \times 3$, or 27 times!

Inefficient swimming technique and poor pool design produce waves. A top-rated swimming pool has gutters that absorb waves. In addition, specially designed lane dividers absorb waves and stop them flowing from one lane to the next.

When an athlete has poor swimming technique, wave drag is likely to increase along with other forms of drag. In events like the famous Hawaiian Iron Man and Iron Woman Triathlons, wave drag caused by the ocean and by other competitors can be a significant form of resistance. Expert swimmers hone their swimming techniques to cut wave drag to a minimum. They also

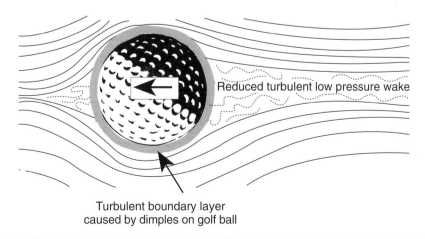

Fig. 6.12. Turbulent flow pattern. At *extremely high* velocities the boundary layer becomes fully turbulent, reducing the size of the low pressure wake. As a result, form drag is reduced.

learn to draft in the wake of a leading swimmer. This simulates the drafting used by cyclists, and in doing this they can swim with less expenditure of energy.

There are two ways of beating wave drag. One is for the athlete to swim under water as long as possible. This technique used to occur in breaststroke and at the start of backstroke races until rule changes restricted how much underwater swimming could occur.

The second method of beating wave drag is hydroplaning. This is a technique in which the pressure the water exerts on the planing surfaces of an object like a speedboat lifts the boat out of the water. The effect is to reduce wave drag and the surface and form drag caused by the water. This "stone-skipping" technique used by speed boats as they hurtle across the surface of the water hardly promotes stability! Proof of this can be found in the high-risk hydroplane races held yearly at Lake Washington near Seattle.

Lift

When an athlete throws a discus, it applies force to the air, and the air reacts by applying force to the discus. The force that the air exerts can be broken down into two separate forces. One acts in the same direction as the airflow. This directly counteracts the implement's forward movement and is the drag force we discussed earlier. The other force acts at right angles to the drag force and is called **lift**. Drag and lift combine to produce a resultant force that most commonly pushes upward and backward, and opposes the motion of the discus. These forces are shown in Figure 6.13.

Experimentation in a wind tunnel with the tilt of the discus relative to the airflow (called the **angle of attack**) indicates that variations in this angle determine how much lift and drag a discus experiences. When the leading edge of the discus is tilted upward as it is in Figure 6.13, air is deflected downward and exerts an equal and opposite pressure upward. This equal and opposite pressure produces the upward lift acting on the discus.

There is a limit on how much the leading edge can be angled upward and still give the discus lift. If the angle is too great, lift disappears and drag increases dramatically causing the discus to

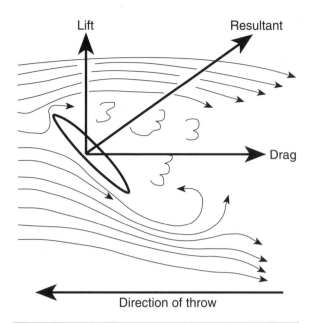

Fig. 6.13. Lift and drag forces combine to form a resultant force.

stall. Figure 6.14a shows a worst-case scenario. A discus thrown in this fashion gets no lift at all and quickly drops to the ground. If the leading edge of the discus is tilted downward, the lift force acts downward. As strange as it may seem, this is still called lift. Lift does not have to be upward though the word "lift" suggests this! Lift can be any direction. In Figure 6.14b the resultant of lift and drag forces acts backward and downward opposing the motion of the discus.

Many factors influence the amount of lift acting not only on a discus but on an athlete as well. Lift is influenced by the shape of the athlete and the athlete's body position, because shape influences airflow patterns as they pass by. The body position assumed by one of the great Norwegian ski jumpers traveling down the ramp is much different from the position they use immediately after takeoff. Accelerating down the ramp, they crouch low with their backs parallel to the ramp. This not only reduces drag but minimizes air pressing against their chests and lifting upward. When they take off, their bodies are extended and angled forward and upward so the angle of attack maximizes lift. Holding this position, lift extends the time that they are in the air and helps to produce their soaring jumps of more than 300 ft (see Figure 6.15).

The faster that a ski jumper flies through the air, the greater the lift force that pushes him upward. This force depends on the ski jumper hold-

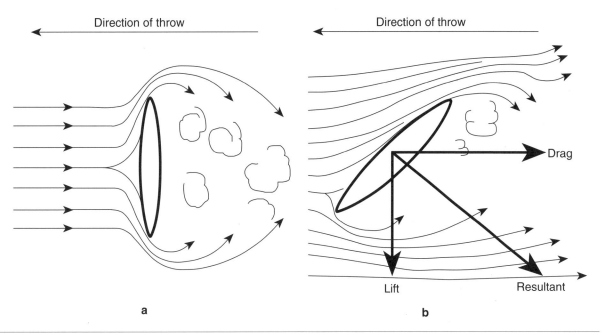

Fig. 6.14.   (a) Discus thrown in this manner gets no lift. (b) Discus thrown with a negative angle of attack generates downward lift.

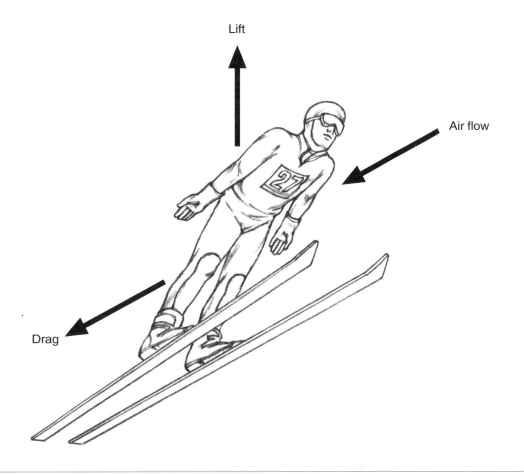

Fig. 6.15.   Lift and drag in a ski jump.

ing an optimal body angle to maximize lift. The jumper must change this angle as he slows in flight. Likewise the size of the surface area that the jumper angles into the air flow also influences lift. If this area is increased, the lifting force is increased in much the same way that a larger wing surface on a plane increases lift. This is why there are specific regulations on the suits that ski jumpers wear. Their one-piece suits must allow a certain amount of air to pass through. Why? Because jumpers had been using suits with material in front that allowed air to pass through and a different material at the back that trapped the air, thereby gaining a lift advantage!

Finally, the consistency of the fluid and its relative motion dramatically influence lift. When air and water are thicker (denser), lift is increased, and the faster the fluid moves by an object, the greater the lift. This means that a water-skier will experience more lift skimming across the ocean than across a freshwater lake. Similarly a ski jumper will get more lift at lower altitudes where the air is more dense than in the thinner air of high altitudes.

The amount of lift that an athlete requires varies according to the demands of the sport. Downhill speed skiers compete to see who can reach the greatest speed (often faster than 130 mph) through a measured section of the course. The last thing these athletes want is lift. Their skis are purposely long and heavy with tips that have hardly any curl so they do not lift off the snow.

Speed skiers fight to keep their upper bodies parallel to the ground. In this way the lift from the upper body is minimal. Their body positions and equipment design are intended to keep them locked onto the snow.

Waterskiing differs from speed skiing because lift is a necessity. Unless the athlete gets lift there is no hope of rising onto the surface of the water. A boat must pull the athlete at an adequate velocity because this helps to produce lift. The faster the boat the more lift. In addition, the athlete angles the tips of the skis more at the start than when traveling on the surface. By doing this, the reaction force from the water combines with the pull of the boat to lift the athlete out of the water and into a skiing position (see Figure 6.16).

Downward lift (and the resultant of drag and lift) is commonly used in auto racing where front and rear spoilers are angled to press the car down onto the road. This improves the friction of the tires with the road surface and gives better traction (see Figure 6.17). Downward lift can also occur during swimming strokes. We discuss this in the next section.

Lift and Drag as Propulsive Forces

Earlier in this chapter we looked at how drag forces oppose the motion of an athlete. In this section we will see that under certain circum-

New Rules Bring Javelins Back to Earth

Until the rules were changed, technicians realized that if a javelin was made "fatter," with very little taper from either end to the grip, it had an increased surface area and got more support from the air. If its center of gravity was shifted back toward the midpoint, the javelin would follow a much flatter and longer trajectory. In the hands of a superb thrower and under perfect wind conditions, a javelin of this type would fly incredible distances. In 1984 Uwe Hohn of East Germany (who held his country's military record for throwing a 21 oz practice grenade over 328 ft) threw such a javelin an incredible 343 ft 10 in. Rule makers flipped! Javelins flying this far would endanger athletes at the other end of the stadium. What did they do? They moved the center of gravity forward and put specific controls on the shape and taper of the javelin. Distances temporarily dropped. Now with talented athletes and improved training techniques, javelin throws are back over 300 ft again (Modified from Wallechinsky, 1991, p. 115).

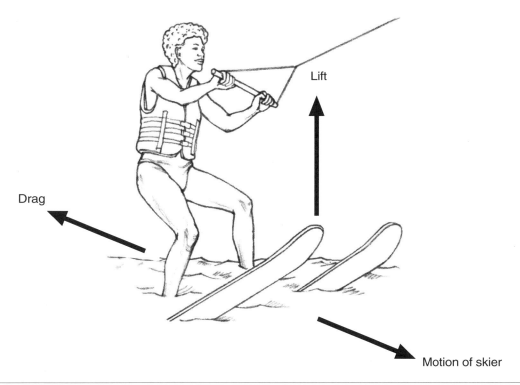

Fig. 6.16.   Lift and drag in water skiing.

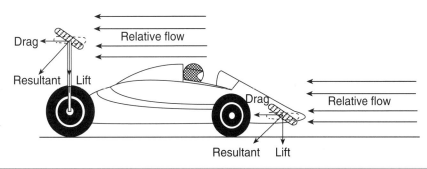

Fig. 6.17.   Lift and the resultant of lift and drag produced by spoilers press a race car down onto the track and improve its traction.
Adapted from Hay and Reid 1988.

stances drag and lift can act as propulsive forces. We'll see how this occurs in the sport of swimming.

If you look at a cross section of an airplane wing, you notice that the underneath side of the wing is fairly flat and the upper side is curved. As the plane moves forward, the curve forces the air flowing over the curved side of the wing to accelerate. The air passing underneath stays at the same speed. Any time that a fluid (in this case the air) speeds up, it exerts less pressure than the same fluid traveling slower. So there is less pressure above the wing than below. The high pressure below the wing forces the wing upward (see Figure 6.18a). The lift produced by the shape of the wing is further enhanced by tilting up the leading edge of the wing (i.e., increasing its angle of attack relative to the air flow) (see Figure 6.18b).

In swimming, athletes purposely shape their hands like the wings of airplanes. By moving them in the appropriate direction through the water, they create lift forces that help propulsion. In addition, by regulating the angle of their hands during the propulsive phases of their stroke, swimmers can select the best angle of attack. This action helps increase lift forces and aids in propulsion.

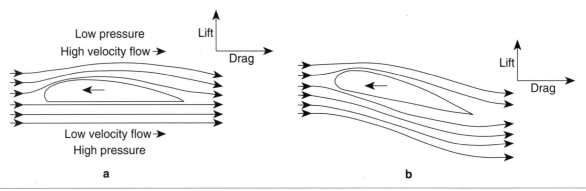

Fig. 6.18.   Lift and drag produced by airflow over an airfoil. (a) High pressure below the wing forces the wing upward. (b) Tilting the leading edge of the wing upward increases lift.
Adapted from Maglischo 1983.

In many ways, a swimmer's hands and feet act like blades of a propeller (which are several wing shapes or airfoils attached to a central hub). When a propeller on a boat spins around, the leading edge of each blade slices into the water. The spin of the propeller makes the water flow toward the trailing edge of the blade. As it passes over the curved upper surface of each blade the water is reduced in pressure and the lift force produced propels the boat forward (see Figure 6.19). In addition, the tilt (or pitch) of the blade deflects water backward.

It's easy for swimmers to simulate the movement of a propeller blade and the manner in which the blade deflects the water. For example, in a sculling action, which swimmers use to tread water, the movement of the arms back and forth

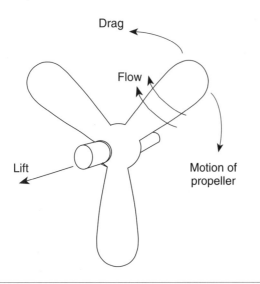

Fig. 6.19.   A propeller is a series of rotating airfoils producing a propulsive lift force.

sideways coupled with variations in pitch (tilt) of the hands, simulates the blade action of a propeller. The sculling action causes the resultant of lift and drag forces to keep the swimmer at the surface of the water (see Figure 6.20, a-b). Sculling is used to great effect in synchronized swimming and in water polo, and a similar sculling action is used in the arm action of the breaststroke (see Figure 6.21). In Figure 6.22, a and b, one phase in the arm action of a crawl stroke is shown. The downward motion of an airfoil (or propeller blade) shown in Figure 6.22a is simulated by the swimmer's hand as it drives downward into the water in Figure 6.22b. The lift produced at this instant in the crawl stroke aids in propelling the swimmer forward.

In the front crawl, variations in the pitch of the hand, coupled with a multidirectional S-shaped arm stroke through the water, produce lift and drag forces that aid propulsion. At certain phases in the stroke, the resultant of lift and drag forces assists in propulsion. Figure 6.23 shows the final phase of the arm pull in the crawl stroke. At this instant in the stroke, the resultant of lift and drag acts as a propulsive force. As with the arm action, the up and down leg beat simulate the upward movement of one propeller blade and the simultaneous downward movement of another. This provides a propulsive lift force that helps push the swimmer forward.

Vortex Propulsion

Recent research suggests that a series of rolling water vortexes created by body and leg actions can assist in propelling a swimmer through the water.

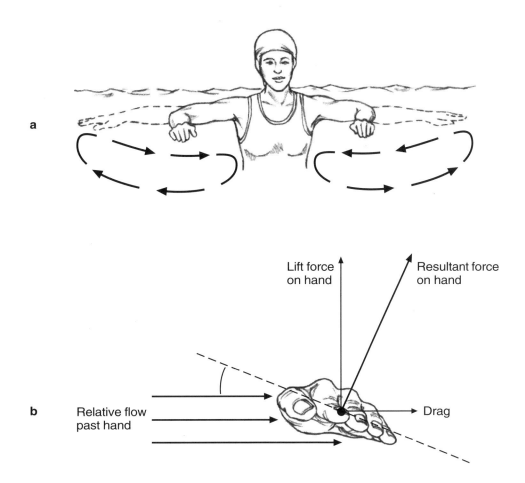

Fig. 6.20. The resultant of lift and drag keeps the sculling swimmer at the surface of the pool. (a) Arm and hand movements of a swimmer treading water and (b) angle of the hand.
Adapted from Kreighbaum and Barthels 1990.

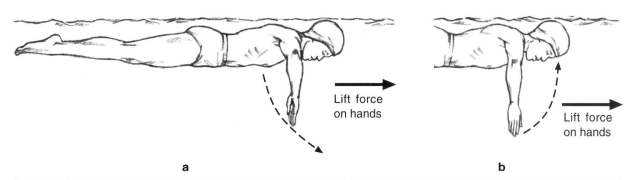

Fig. 6.21. Propulsion from the sideways blading action of the swimmer's hands in the breaststroke. (a) Outward blading of the hands and (b) inward blading of the hands. For both, the lift force that is generated aids in propulsion.
Adapted from Kreighbaum and Barthels 1990.

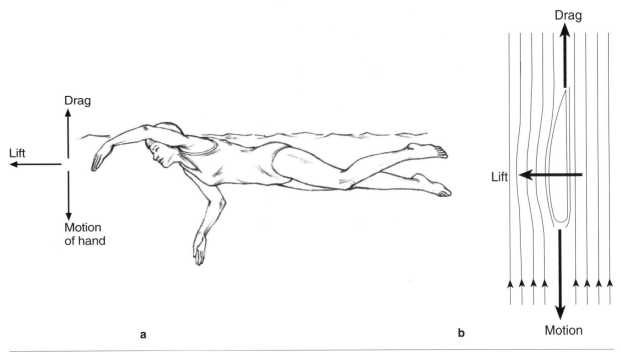

Fig. 6.22. The downward motion of the crawl swimmer's hand produces propulsive lift.

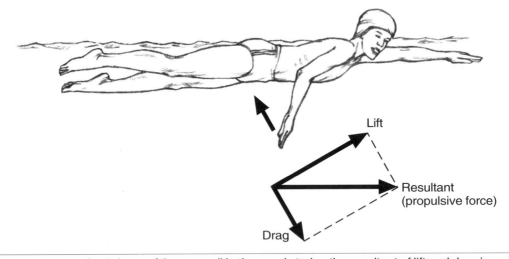

Fig. 6.23. In the final phase of the arm pull in the crawl stroke, the resultant of lift and drag is a propulsive force.

A **vortex** is a mass of swirling fluid, in this case, water. In the butterfly stroke a swimmer, like Olympic champion Pablo Morales, simulates the undulating body motion of a fish, in particular, the dolphin. Vortexes (i.e., swirls of water) are produced by the undulating action (see Figure 6.24). Modern research suggests that the vortexes not only cancel drag but also produce a highly efficient form of jet propulsion (i.e., a form of hydrodynamic push) that shoves fish and swimmer along. Efforts are now being made to design ar-

ticulated (i.e., multijointed) submarines that harness this highly efficient undulating motion!

The Magnus Effect

The **Magnus effect** is a lift force that has tremendous importance in all sports in which athletes want to bend the flight of a ball. You see the Magnus effect at work in the curved flight path of balls thrown, hit, or kicked with a spin. Golfers, baseball pitchers, soccer players, tennis, and

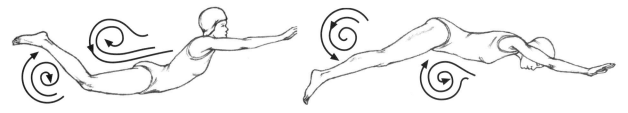

Fig. 6.24.   Vortex propulsion in the butterfly.

table tennis players all employ the Magnus effect to curve the flight path of the ball. In particular the game of baseball is made more fascinating by the Magnus effect. The ability of a pitcher to throw curveballs, sliders, screwballs, and mix in knuckleballs which have very little spin, and then for a batter to hit these pitches, is the essence of baseball!

The Magnus effect operates in the following manner. As a spinning ball moves through the air, it spins a boundary layer of air that clings to its surface as it travels along. On one side of the ball the boundary layer of air collides with air passing by. The collision causes the air to decelerate and this creates a high pressure area. On the opposing side, the boundary layer is moving in the same direction as the air passing by, so there is no collision and the air collectively moves faster. This sets up a low pressure area. The pressure differential, high on one side and low on the other, creates a lift force that causes the ball to move in the direction of the pressure differential (i.e., from high to low) (see Figure 6.25).

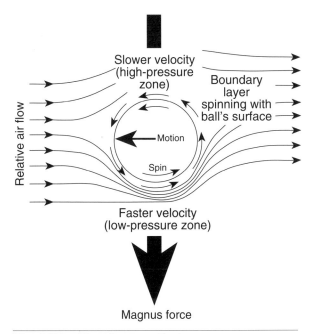

Fig. 6.25.   The Magnus effect.

The Magnus effect can be applied in any direction, and in this way an athlete can create backspin, topspin, and side spin. A soccer player like the great Pelé was well known for the way he used his "banana kicks" (i.e., the Magnus effect) to curve free kicks and corner kicks around defenders and into the goal mouth (see Figure 6.26). Tennis players and volleyball players use the Magnus effect when they apply topspin to make the ball drop suddenly while in flight. Elite golfers use the Magnus effect to produce their controlled hooks, draws, and fades, and the weekend hacker unwittingly applies spin and uses the Magnus effect to slice the ball off to the left and right.

The Magnus effect can combine with the force of gravity or fight against gravity. A topspin combines with gravity's downward pull, and this is why you'll see Pete Sampras and Andre Agassi's topspin forehands arcing viciously over the net and down toward the court. A backspin, on the other hand, fights against gravity. Steffi Graf knows that a backspin lob from her opponent fights gravity's downward pull and will "hang" in the air. Time in the air means extra time to get to the ball.

In golf a club like an 8 or 9 iron is steeply angled to give the ball tremendous backspin. The spin helps the ball to fight gravity and gives it terrific lift, plus the possibility of stopping dead when it lands. In baseball the raised stitches on the ball produce the same effect as dimples on a golf ball. The seams grab a thick boundary layer and in this way a spinning baseball gets plenty of help from the Magnus effect. Pitchers throw curveballs with a powerful snapping action of the wrist. This gives the ball terrific spin. The more spin, the greater the Magnus effect, and the more the curve. A right-handed pitcher like Nolan Ryan combined topspin and side spin so the ball not only dropped but also moved laterally across the plate. Spin, gravity, and drag forces all worked together to produce this effect (see Figure 6.27).

What happens when there is hardly any spin put on a baseball? A pitch with a slight spin is

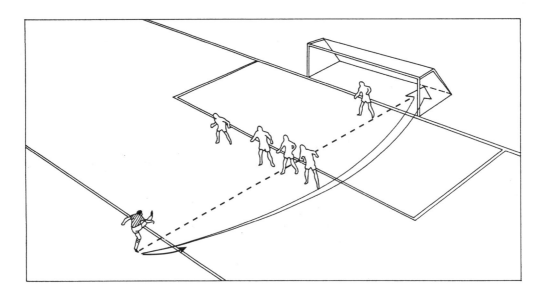

Fig. 6.26. The Magnus effect in a soccer free kick.
Reprinted from Hall 1995.

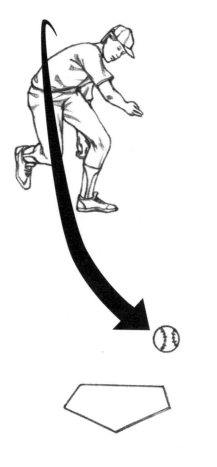

Fig. 6.27. A curve ball moves down and laterally across the plate.

called a knuckleball, and in volleyball a serve with hardly any spin is a floater. The characteristics of a knuckleball and a floater can be summed up in one word: unpredictability. In baseball not even the pitcher knows for sure where the ball is going to end up. Both the knuckleball and floater shift and flutter around in flight. It is this erratic movement that is so confusing to the batter in baseball and to the receiver in volleyball. A pitcher gives a knuckleball a lobbing or pushing release, so it is traveling slowly and maybe spins for one full revolution by the time it reaches the batter. During flight air flowing past at one instant grabs at the seams and at another instant contacts the smooth surfaces of the ball. The ball may go straight for a while, then it suddenly veers to the right or the left and possibly back again. Pitchers have learned that a ball released at a certain speed will start by having a regular flight pattern. Halfway to the plate the ball slows down to a critical level. At this point drag forces build up dramatically and the ball suddenly drops. All this is meant to confuse the batter. But if the pitcher makes the error of throwing the ball with too much spin or too much speed, the knuckleball becomes an easy target for the batter.

It is well known that greasing, cutting, scuffing, or wetting the surface of the ball can produce the strange antics of the knuckleball. A ball that has been treated in this manner will act like a knuckleball but at a faster speed. In a game that the pitcher already dominates, these actions gave too much advantage to the pitcher and as a result have been outlawed.

All the pitches thrown in baseball are affected in one way or another by environmental conditions. As a generalization, dense air helps to move the ball around, whereas thin air at high altitude makes it easy for the ball to go faster. Knuckleballs become less deceptive at high altitude and as temperature rises. In these conditions, the game belongs to the slugger and the fastball pitcher!

SUMMARY

1. An athlete or object moving through a fluid is affected by hydrostatic pressure (exerted by the weight of a fluid), buoyancy (the force opposing gravity that acts on objects partially or totally immersed in a fluid), drag (the force opposing motion through a fluid), and lift (the force acting perpendicularly to motion that deflects an object from its original pathway).

2. The pressure that the atmosphere exerts on the earth's surface is 14.7 psi. An increase in altitude decreases this pressure progressively.

3. The pressure exerted by water increases with depth. In the ocean, pressure is increased approximately one atmosphere (14.7 psi) for every 33 ft of depth.

4. The buoyant force acting on an athlete is equal to the weight of the fluid that the athlete's body displaces when immersed in the fluid.

5. The center of buoyancy is the place where the buoyant force concentrates its upward thrust on an object immersed in a fluid. The center of buoyancy is usually positioned higher on an athlete's body than is the athlete's center of gravity.

6. Atmospheric pressure, temperature, and the contents of air or water affect how the water and air act: The more dense or viscous a fluid, the greater the frictional forces acting on an athlete or an object immersed in that fluid.

7. The frictional forces occurring when an object or athlete moves through a fluid are the same as when fluids flow at the same velocity past the object or the athlete.

8. Laminar flow, which is smooth and regular, occurs around an object when fluid flow is slow. Turbulent flow, which is disturbed and rough, occurs at high velocities. Turbulent flow generates more drag than laminar flow.

9. The three types of drag are surface drag, form drag, and wave drag.

10. Surface drag is also called skin friction or viscous drag. The amount of surface drag is determined by the relative motion of object and fluid, the area of surface exposed to the flow, the roughness of the object's surface, and the fluid viscosity.

11. Form drag is also called shape drag or pressure drag. The amount of form drag is determined by the relative motion of object and fluid, the pressure differential between the leading and trailing edges of the object, and the amount of surface acting at right angles to the flow.

12. Wave drag occurs at the interface between water and air. The amount of wave drag is determined by the relative velocity with which the object and wave meet, the surface area of the object acting at right angles to the wave, and the fluid viscosity.

13. At high velocities turbulent flow produces a low pressure wake acting to the rear of an object. This low pressure area is used in sport for drafting or slipstreaming.

14. Balls moving through the air suffer from form and surface drag. The lower pressure wake to the rear of the ball is reduced by increasing the surface drag: An increase in surface drag can help decrease the ball's form drag.

15. Athletes and objects are affected by lift forces that depend on the relative motion of the object and the fluid, the angle of the object relative to the flow of the fluid, the size of the surface area angled into the fluid flow, and the nature of the fluid.

16. Swimmers angle their hands and feet to create lift, which can act as a propulsive force. At certain phases in the hand and leg actions of a swimmer, the resultant of lift and drag forces can act as a propulsive force.

17. Swirling water, called vortexes, is produced by the undulating motion of a fish—or of an athlete performing the dolphin leg kick. Vortexes can reduce drag and can assist in propulsion.

18. A spinning object (e.g., a ball) traveling through the air builds up high pressure on the side spinning into the airflow. Low pressure occurs on the side spinning *with* the airflow. The ball is deflected from high pressure to low pressure. This phenomenon is called the Magnus effect.

REVIEW QUESTIONS

1. A scuba diver mistakenly holds his breath on the way to the surface from 66 ft. How many lungsful of air will a single lungful become when the diver reaches the surface?

2. A muscular, lean gymnast weighing 100 lb and an obese sumo wrestler weighing 400 lb jump into a swimming pool. Why is the obese sumo wrestler more likely to float?

3. The world record for pedaling a bike behind a pace vehicle is held by John Howard of the United States at 150-plus mph! Why was it unnecessary for John and his bike to be streamlined?

4. Why can recumbent cyclists covered in an aerodynamic shell cycle faster than the world's best sprint cyclists?

5. What characteristics of an airfoil cause lift to occur?

6. How does the Magnus effect deflect a spinning ball?

PART TWO

Putting Your Knowledge of Mechanics to Work

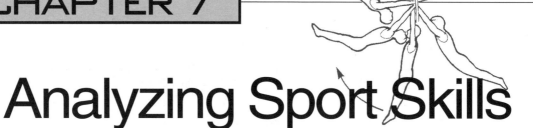

CHAPTER 7

Analyzing Sport Skills

When you finish reading this chapter, you should be able to explain

- how to determine skill objectives;

- how knowing the special characteristics of a skill can help you analyze athletic performance;

- what you gain from an analysis of the performances of top-flight athletes;

- how to divide a skill into phases and key elements; and

- how to use your knowledge of mechanics in the analysis of a skill and the correction of errors.

Chapters 7 and 8 are closely linked and will show you how to put your knowledge of sport mechanics to work. Here you'll find advice on how to break a skill into smaller parts. This process will make it easier when you critically observe your athlete's performance. Chapter 8 gives you examples of observation techniques and teaches you how to select errors that need correcting.

One of the greatest challenges you'll face if you coach is watching your athlete perform and deciding which aspect of the skill needs correction. If you don't have a well-planned approach, you're likely to be overwhelmed by the complexity and speed of the skill you are trying to analyze. You'll not know what aspect of the skill to

look at, or what error to correct first. You may see so many errors at once that you throw your hands up in the air, and in desperation give vague coaching tips like "hit harder," or "be more aggressive!" Advice like this is of little assistance to your athlete. What you need to do is gather background information about the skill before you start, and come to each coaching session with a precise plan to guide your observation, your analysis, and the correction of errors. If you understand the mechanics inherent in the technique of the skill your athlete is performing and you know how to go after major errors, your athlete benefits immensely and quickly improves in performance.

The information that you need before you start correcting errors is in this chapter in a series of steps:

Step 1. Determine the Objectives of the Skill

Step 2. Note Any Special Characteristics of the Skill

Step 3. Study Top-Flight Performances of the Skill

Step 4. Divide the Skill Into Phases

Step 5. Divide Each Phase Into Key Elements

Step 6. Understand the Mechanical Reasons Each Key Element Is Performed as It Is

If you work your way through each step, you'll learn how to break a skill into important parts (or phases), and you'll know how to use your knowledge of sport mechanics when you analyze each phase. You'll find out how much easier it is to analyze each phase of a skill rather than concentrating on the total skill, then trying to recollect what happened!

Don't feel that you must go through each step *every time* you teach a skill. Once you have read this chapter, you'll understand what information you need, and with a little practice, you'll find that you can carry out most of the steps in your head. To begin with, however, write down on a clipboard the information that's required. Then take this material with you and use it as a guide during your coaching sessions.

Step 1. Determine the Objectives of the Skill

The rules of the sport and the conditions that exist when a sport skill is performed determine **skill objectives**. You'll find that most skills have more than one objective. It's good to be aware of these objectives because they determine the technique and mechanics that your athlete must use to perform the skill successfully. Let's look at some sport skills and see what we mean by skill objectives.

The dominant objective for your athlete competing in the discus event is to throw the implement as far as possible. The farther the discus travels, the better. However, accuracy of flight is an important objective as well because the discus has to land within a sector. The distance thrown is discounted if the discus lands outside the sector lines. The discus can even land within the sector lines, but if the thrower loses balance and falls out of the ring, the throw is declared invalid.

The objectives of distance and accuracy determine what mechanical principles to keep in mind when you coach your athlete in the discus. The overriding importance of distance tells you that the dominant mechanical objective in the event is maximum velocity at release. This means you will concentrate on teaching your athlete how to have the discus leave her hand as fast as possible.

How the discus leaves your athlete's hand and how it spins determine its flight characteristics and its distance. So you cannot forget that an optimal spin and trajectory are important objectives too. You also have to remember that the body positions your athlete uses during the throw influence the distance and flight of the discus and your athlete's stability after the discus is released. It would be a tragedy if every throw was a world record distance but declared a foul because your athlete fell out the front of the ring!

In a volleyball spike, your athlete has to jump high enough to strike the ball over, around, or off the blockers. The prime objective of a spike is to get the ball to hit the floor in the opponent's court (see Figure 7.1). To achieve this objective, jumping ability and timing are tremendously important, and so is accuracy in directing the ball. In addition, your athlete has to take care not to contact the net. Keep these objectives in mind when you coach spiking skills. Work on the mechanics of the approach, the jump, the spiking action, and then control of the body after the ball has left your athlete's hand.

Compare the objectives of the volleyball spike with those required of a high jumper. Height is obviously a prime objective in high jump just as it is in a volleyball spike. However, a high jumper is also required to cross a bar—an objective not required of a volleyball player. So a high jumper has to jump both vertically and horizontally, then rotate in the air to get into a good bar clearance position. It's no use producing great height by itself or having a good bar clearance technique if your athlete cannot get up into the air!

In weight lifting, the prime objective is to hoist a barbell to arm's length above the head. A secondary objective is to have control over the bar-

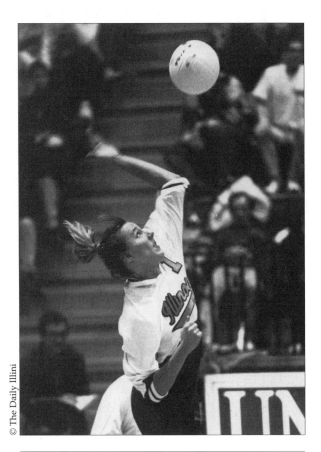

Fig. 7.1. The objectives of a volleyball spike are (a) to either land the ball in the opponent's court or deflect it off an opponent's block so it goes out-of-bounds; (b) to avoid contacting the net; (c) to avoid landing with one or both feet in the opponent's court.

bell once it's in this position. This second criterion is necessary for the judges to pass the lift. Even though the barbell must be held steady for a relatively short time, control and stability are still important objectives and have to be taught for your athlete to achieve success in this skill.

Whatever sport you coach, whether it is an individual or team sport, it is important that you are aware of *all* the objectives required of each skill. If you coach to satisfy one objective and forget or deemphasize another, you'll limit the success of your athlete. What use is it if a water polo player learns to fire the ball at phenomenal velocity if no emphasis is placed on controlling and directing the path of the ball? Similarly, what use is it if you teach a diver how to get great height and spin, if the diver then hits the board on the way down or the entry into the water is a disaster? So be aware of all the objectives required by a skill, and remember that all these objectives play a part in determining the technique that you teach your athlete.

Step 2. Note Any Special Characteristics of the Skill

Sport skills can be divided into different types based on (a) the *manner* in which your athlete performs the skill, and (b) the *conditions* under which your athlete performs the skill. Both manner and conditions are interrelated and both dramatically influence the methods you will use when you coach. For example, if you consider just the manner in which skills are performed, you'll see that some skills are performed once, then a totally different action occurs next. Other skills are different because they repeat sequentially. These two types can be called *nonrepetitive* and *repetitive* skills.

The conditions under which athletes perform skills also differ considerably. Some conditions are controlled and *predictable*. You know what the conditions are going to be like before the competition starts. Other conditions vary considerably and are *unpredictable*, and it's difficult to know what they'll be like when the competition begins.

Let's first look at nonrepetitive and repetitive skills and then at predictable and unpredictable conditions.

Nonrepetitive Skills

Nonrepetitive skills are often called "discrete" skills in that they have a definite beginning and an end—even though they can be repeated more than once in a sporting situation. There are many examples, such as a tower dive, a shot put, or a bunt in baseball. Skills like these do not repeat in sequence. Instead some other action occurs immediately afterward. If your athlete is a diver, she'll land in the pool, climb out, and wait for her turn in the next round of dives. A similar situation occurs for the shot-putter, who after throwing must wait for other competitors to complete their throw before he can perform again. The baseball player follows a bunt with a totally different action. In most cases it's a sprint to first base.

You'll find that you can easily teach nonrepetitive skills as separate entities. Once the skill has been well taught, you add some other skill or action to lead into it, or to lead out of it, similar to the baseball player bunting and sprinting to first base or a gymnast performing a handspring followed by a dive-roll.

Nonrepetitive Skills in Sequence

Frequently the momentum generated in one nonrepetitive skill will carry over and assist in beginning another nonrepetitive skill. A young gymnast builds a floor exercise routine in this manner. A handspring may join a front somersault, and the somersault leads into another skill. Similarly, a triple jumper hops, steps, and finally jumps. The three jumps differ, yet the skill of triple jumping depends on the synchronization of all three skills. For an excellent distance, the hop must contribute to the step, and the step to the jump (see Figure 7.2).

When you coach nonrepetitive or discrete skills in sequence, it's a good idea to teach each skill separately. Then teach your athlete to adapt to the rhythm pattern and changes that occur when two or three skills are performed in sequence. Be aware that two or three skills in sequence present additional difficulties for your athlete. Novice triple jumpers frequently perform an immense hop only to collapse at the end of it and have nothing left for the step or the jump. There is no balanced effort or flow from the hop to the step and finally to the jump.

In gymnastics a young athlete can learn to perform a back somersault by itself. Then you can teach her to perform a round-off that leads into the back somersault. If correctly performed, the round-off makes the performance of a back somersault easier. Performed poorly, the round-off positions the gymnast incorrectly for the takeoff into the back somersault. This makes it difficult for the gymnast to get around and safely complete the somersault.

Repetitive Skills

Repetitive skills are those that have a cyclic, continuous nature. For example, the actions that make up the movement pattern of sprinting repeat continuously during the race. This repetitive, continuous feature occurs in many sports such as race-walking, cycling, swimming, speed skating, and cross-country skiing.

The most important aspect of repetitive skills is that one complete cycle of the skill immedi-

ately leads into the next. This means that a follow-through (which slows down and dissipates energy in a nonrepetitive skill) becomes a recovery in a repetitive skill and is essential for maintaining continuity and rhythm.

In competitive swimming, athletes aim for a fast arm recovery when they perform their strokes. The arms complete their pull in the water, then quickly cycle forward into the next propulsive action. There is no braking action, or dissipation of energy as occurs in the follow-through of a discus or a javelin throw. Like the cyclist who wishes to keep the pedals spinning at a high rate, the competitive swimmer wishes to do the same thing with the arms after each arm pull (see Figure 7.3).

Repetitive skills are frequently taught to young athletes in much the same way as discrete nonrepetitive skills. The crawl stroke is first broken into leg action, arm action, and breathing. These components of the stroke are taught separately and then molded together to build the complete skill. The number of repeats or cycles of the total skill is progressively increased as the athlete's ability improves.

Skills Performed in Predictable Environments

Many skills are performed in a precise predictable environment. Frequently these types of skills are described as **closed skills**. In this situation your athlete can get on with the job of performing the skill without having to make quick decisions because of a sudden change in conditions. A clean and jerk in weight lifting and the skills in a synchronized swimming routine are examples. The fact that your athlete can concentrate on the lift or on the skills in the synchronized swimming routine without worrying about the actions of opposing players, or changes in weather conditions, makes practice sessions easier for you to plan and training easier for your athlete.

Skills Performed in Unpredictable Environments

Many sport skills are performed in an unpredictable environment. These skills are often described as **open skills**. The most frequent cause of the unpredictable environment is the presence of opposition whose prime purpose is to make your athlete fail in whatever he or she is trying to do.

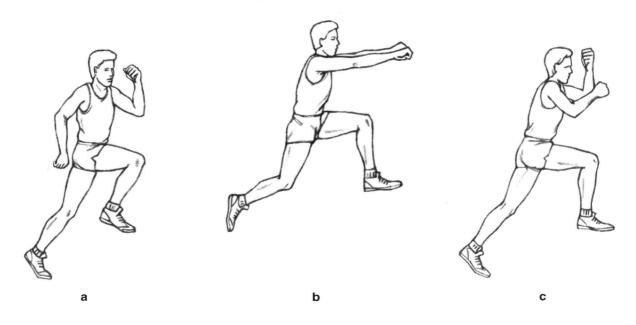

a   b   c

Fig. 7.2.   The triple jump is an example of three discrete skills in sequence: the hop, the step, and the jump.

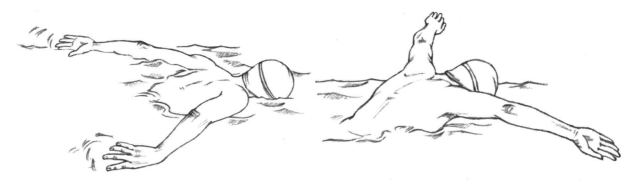

Fig. 7.3.   Swimming strokes are examples of cyclic, repetitive skills in which the recovery of the arms and legs leads into the next propulsive phase.

Consequently, your athlete has to respond according to the conditions that occur in any instant during the competition. In baseball, your batter has to respond (in less than 1/2 sec!) to whatever pitch is thrown. Your volleyball player has to be able to respond according to the serve that comes over the net. Her response is going to be different for a floater serve than a fast topspin spike serve. In freestyle wrestling and judo, your athlete must attack or defend according to the maneuvers of the opponent. In soccer, a goalkeeper must react according to the maneuvers and shot fired by an attacking player.

Besides opposition, wind, waves, rain, sun, and varying field and court conditions can cause uncertainty and unpredictability. A surfer has to assess the nature of the wave and perform surfing skills accordingly. Each wave has to be considered individually when it occurs, and the surfer has to develop an ability to cope with these conditions. The variability that exists in all the sports we've mentioned, from baseball to wrestling, forces your athlete to make sudden decisions and to perform skills at varying velocities. This means that the ability to judge the situation and to react quickly is important.

When you coach open skills, which are performed in unpredictable conditions, begin by making the situation as predictable as possible. For example, wrestlers work repeatedly on the same defensive maneuver against an opponent who is required to repeat the attacking move. In

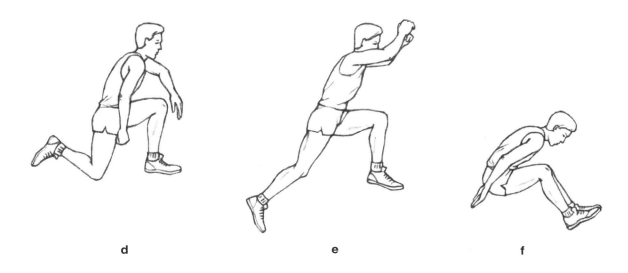

d   e   f

baseball and tennis, players face balls fired repeatedly and predictably from pitching and serving machines, and in rugby, football, and field hockey, athletes practice set plays without opposition. Then other team members work as opposition and the same plays are repeated. In this way the mechanics of a particular skill are practiced in a predictable situation until the quality of the skill performance is good. Then more unpredictability is introduced.

The speed with which unpredictability is introduced depends on many factors, one of the most important being the speed with which the athlete learns the required skill. Many coaches like to move quickly to unpredictable situations. Others mix up drills so that the athlete learns rapidly how to judge "what should be done" in some drills. In other drills the athlete works on a particular skill repeatedly under predictable conditions.

Step 3. Study Top-Flight Performances of the Skill

When you watch top-class athletes perform a skill, you get a picture of the speed, rhythm, power, body positions, and other characteristics that make up a quality performance. This helps you understand the basic movement patterns in the technique of the skill you intend to coach. It's

a good idea to use a video camera and tape these performances from various angles. Then you can watch the skill repeatedly at normal speed and in slow motion. You'll soon notice that, in spite of differences in body type, the techniques top athletes use all show common features. Elite golfers shift their body weight and rotate their hips in much the same way. Great throwers in track and field use similar throwing positions and activate their muscles in a similar sequence. Top-class divers use a similar hurdle step and drive up off the springboard with similar arm and leg actions. These identical features exist because top class athletes have been coached to use good mechanics. Their coaches have taught them to use actions in their performances that produce the optimal force, velocity, spin, and so forth, required by the skill.

As you progress through steps 4, 5, and 6 in this chapter, you'll get used to associating mechanical principles with technique. You'll notice that you use your knowledge of mechanics when you look at an elite performance. You'll be able to say to yourself, "I understand the mechanical reasons Nancy Lopez and Pat Bradley shift their weight and rotate their hips when they drive a golf ball, and I understand why their arms are extended when the club head contacts the ball." You'll realize that these technical features are necessary actions that must be taught to all young golfers irrespective of their shape, size, and build. The same principles apply to the skills of any sport. Elite performers use good technique based on sound mechanics and so provide you with a model on which to base your coaching.

Step 4. Divide the Skill Into Phases

Your next task is to divide the skill you're interested in coaching into phases. This process is important because it makes your job much easier when you look for errors in your athlete's performance. Quite simply, it stops you from becoming confused by trying to watch too much of the skill at the same time.

Most skills consist of several phases. A **phase** is a connected group of movements that appear to stand on their own and that your athlete joins together in the performance of the total skill. Many skills, for example, can be broken down into the following four phases:

1. Preparatory Movements and Mental Set
2. Wind-Up (or Backswing)
3. Force-Producing Movements
4. Follow-Through (or Recovery)

If you look at a golf swing, a slap shot in hockey, or a baseball pitch, the preparatory movements and mental set are the first phase in the skill. The windup (or backswing) is the second phase. These are followed by the third phase, which includes the force-producing movements. The skill is completed by a fourth phase, which is the follow-through (see Figure 7.4). Each phase, starting from the preparatory movements and mental set, leads into and influences the next phase in line like a chain reaction. This common characteristic tells you that errors occurring during an early phase of a skill are bound to affect all the phases that follow. So when something goes wrong at the end of a skill, you'll examine not only the last phase but also earlier phases to see if the root of the problem lies there. For example, if a golfer makes an error in setting up and addressing the ball, or performs the backswing incorrectly, the effect of

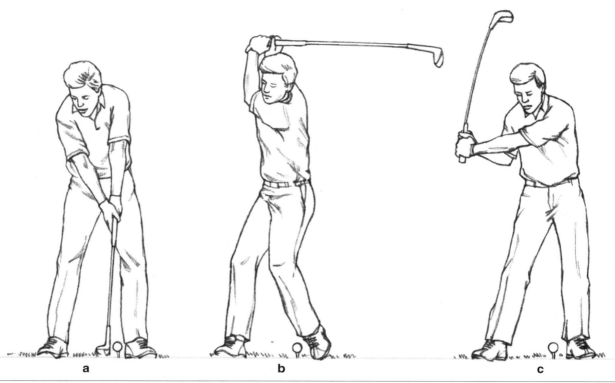

a   b   c

Fig. 7.4. Phases of a golf drive are the (a) preparatory movements and mental set, (b) backswing, (c and d) force-producing movements, and (e and f) follow-through.

Sport Mechanics Facilitate Olympic Win

Valeri Borzov of the former Soviet Union won the 100 and 200 m in the 1972 Olympic Games. Commenting on Borzov's preparation, coach Valentin Petrovsky said, "We began with a search for the most up-to-date model of sprinting. We studied slow motion films of leading world-class sprinters both past and present. We figured out the best angle of thrust and body position and went into a whole number of minor details. When the mathematical equivalent of a runner was worked out and given a scientific basis, we began testing our calculations in practice. It was subtle work, which could be compared to the training of a ballerina."

(Adopted and modified from Wallechinsky, 1991, p. 11, *The Complete Book of the Olympics*).

the error carries into the remaining parts of the drive, and of course, into the flight of the ball. Don't be deceived by thinking that all errors have their cause in the phase in which they occur. Check out earlier phases. Frequently you'll find the problem lies there!

Let's look at each phase individually and see what specific contributions they make toward the performance of the total skill.

Preparatory Movements and Mental Set

These are the movements and the mental processes that your athlete goes through when setting up and getting ready to perform. The golfer takes up a stance and addresses the ball. The tennis player gets herself ready to serve and mentally decides where to direct the serve. In some

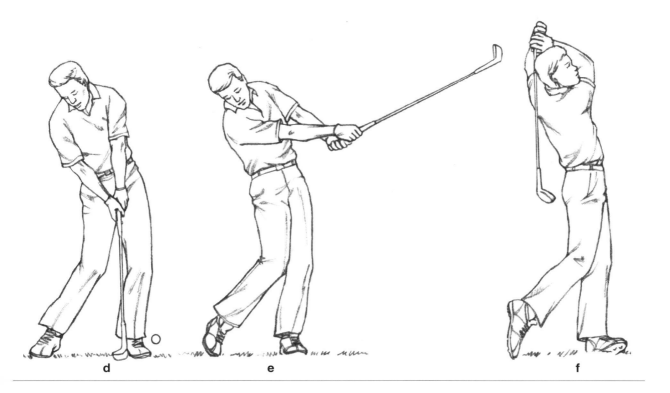

d   e   f positions, such as an offensive lineman preparatory stance, your athlete will crouch with his muscles in a static-stretch position. When the ball is snapped, his muscles respond with an explosive thrusting motion that immediately leads into the next phase of the skill.

In cyclic, repetitive skills there can be a preparatory phase at the start of the skill. Thereafter they normally don't occur. For example, if you coach a butterfly swimmer you don't establish a static stance before each propulsive action. Your athlete flows immediately from each arm pull and leg beat into the next.

Windup (or Backswing)

Many skills use a **windup** or a backswing. These movements stretch your athlete's muscles and establish a position from which your athlete can apply force over a long distance or time frame. Examples are the rotary windup of a discus thrower, a backswing in golf and baseball, and the backward extension of a javelin thrower's arm. In a tennis serve and volleyball spike, the dropping back of the hitting arm to the rear of an athlete's body fulfills a similar purpose to that of a thrower. In kayaking, the forward reach of the paddler before thrusting the blade in the water acts like a windup or backswing.

Force-Producing Movements

Force-producing movements are the specific actions that your athlete uses to generate force. They usually involve the athlete's whole body, and may include a run-up, but in finer, more discrete actions (like archery, or throwing a dart in a darts competition), they may only require the use of the arm and shoulder muscles and minimally involve the muscles of the rest of the body.

Force-producing actions are tremendously important in creating the desired effect in a skill. Your athlete's muscles have to apply force in the correct amount, over the correct range and time period, and in the correct sequence. You'll find that force-producing actions come in many types. They include such sequential actions as the run-up, pull, and push of the pole-vaulter, the body extension and arm flexion of the rower, the rotating spins and throwing actions of the hammer thrower and discus thrower, and the run-up, takeoff, and arm actions involved in a basketball layup. In contrast, in a power lifter's dead lift, the force-producing actions occur almost simul-taneously, with the athlete's leg, back, arms, and shoulder muscles pulling at the same time.

In all skills an important and critical instant in time occurs at the end of the force-producing movements. It happens when a baseball is struck, a takeoff occurs, or an implement is released. At this instant the direction of force is set and force is applied by the athlete. At this point there is nothing more that the athlete can do to upgrade the skill.

Follow-Through (or Recovery)

Follow-through and recovery actions are those actions that occur immediately after the force-producing motions are complete. In throwing skills, the implement has been released, and in hitting skills, the impact has been made. In many skills it is impossible and even dangerous for your athlete to come to a complete stop immediately after the force-producing actions have occurred. The momentum generated causes your athlete's limbs to continue along their original pathway. The follow-through acts to safely dissipate the force of these actions.

In skills in which the movement pattern is repeated in a continuous cyclic fashion, such as in a swimming stroke, the recovery of the arms leads quickly to the next repetition of the arm pull. In these cyclic, repetitious skills, momentum and rhythm are an essential part of the cadence of the complete skill. The recovery actions have the task of helping to maintain balance and continuity of motion. In addition to the swimming stroke, other examples are the leg and arm recovery in sprinting, skating, and cross-country skiing.

Step 5. Divide Each Phase Into Key Elements

When you have chosen the most important phases of a skill, direct your attention toward the task of dividing each phase into its **key elements**. Key elements are distinct actions that join to make up a phase. Using the analogy of a building—try to view a skill as a building that you are erecting. Phases are the walls of your building, and the key elements are the bricks you use to make each wall.

How do you choose key elements? Select key elements as distinct actions that are essential to the success of each phase in the skill (i.e., the same way that phases are essential to the success of the skill!). A windup phase will have its key elements, just as the force-producing phase, and likewise the follow-through.

Here are some examples of key elements. We haven't given you every key element that exists in the phases we've chosen, but we've selected examples to give you an idea of what key elements are! You'll see these key elements in the techniques used by all top-flight athletes. Why? Because these key elements are essential in good technique and contribute mechanically toward the success of the skill. Without them your athlete could not produce an optimal performance.

- In the force-producing phase of a golf drive, your athlete shifts her body weight to the rear foot and from the rear to the forward foot. Your athlete rotates her hips into the drive and has extended arms when the club contacts the ball. *Key elements*: Weight shift, hip rotation, arm extension.

- In the force-producing phase of a javelin throw, your athlete runs up, leans back, and steps forward into a wide throwing position. The athlete then rotates the hips and chest toward the direction of throw. Simultaneously the athlete shifts her body weight from the rear to the forward leg (see Figure 9.4). *Key elements*: Run-up, backward lean, wide throwing position, hip and chest rotation, weight shift.

- In a high jump run-up, which is part of the force-producing phase of a high jump, your athlete leans into the curve of the run-up. At the completion of the run-up your athlete leans back and lowers her center of gravity when stepping into the takeoff position. The arms are positioned to the rear of her body in preparation for swinging forward and upward at takeoff. *Key elements*: Backward lean, lowering of the center of gravity, arms to the rear of the body (see Figure 9.3).

- In a football punt, after stepping forward with the supporting foot, your athlete swings the kicking leg through a long arc. The kicking leg, which starts partially flexed, is fully extended on contact with the ball. Your athlete simultaneously shifts his body weight forward and upward into the punt. The arms, which have fed the ball onto the kicking foot, are extended sideways to maintain balance. *Key elements*: Extended base, weight shift, long kicking arc, leg extension, arm extension (see Figure 9.6).

Remember that there are more key elements in each skill discussed above, and that the sequence in which these elements is performed is an important element in itself! In some phases of a skill, key elements are performed almost simultaneously. In other situations there is a definite flow from one to the next. With practice and careful observation of elite performances, you will be able to pick out *all* the key elements for each phase of a skill and understand the timing of their performance. The next job you have is to understand the mechanical reasons key elements exist and what purpose they serve. This is your next step.

Step 6. Understand the Mechanical Reasons Each Key Element Is Performed as It Is

This is a tremendously important step in your sequence. Chapters 3 through 7 have shown you how mechanics form the foundation of all sport techniques. All the fundamental actions an athlete makes in his or her technique are founded on mechanical principles. In other words, technique is based on mechanical laws! So once you've picked out the key elements in the skill you are analyzing, you have to understand the mechanical purposes behind each element. You must be able to answer questions of the following nature with responses like the ones listed below:

"Why cock and uncock the wrists during a golf drive?"

Cocking and uncocking the wrists during a golf drive causes the golfer's arms and club to simulate the whiplash or flail-like action of the high-speed tip segments of a whip. When the wrists are cocked and uncocked they act as an additional axis around which the club can rotate. The velocity developed from the swing (and length) of the golfer's arms is multiplied along the length of the club shaft. Without the cocking and uncocking action, the arms and club move as a fixed unit. This would not allow the head of the club to reach optimal velocity (see Figure 7.4).

"Why is it important for an athlete to rotate the hips and thrust them ahead of the upper body during a golf drive, shot put, discus, or javelin throw?"

Rotating the hips ahead of the upper body and toward the direction of throw serves three purposes:

1. It shifts the athlete's body mass in the proper direction (i.e., toward the direction that the golf ball, discus, shot, and javelin will be accelerated). This action extends the distance and time over which the athlete applies force.

2. The rotation of the hips acts as an important link in the sequential acceleration of the athlete's body segments. The movement of the athlete's legs and hips toward the direction of throw (and golf drive) simulates swinging a whip handle ahead of the rest of the whip so the tip of the whip will crack!

3. The rotation of the hips stretches the muscles of the abdomen and chest so that they pull the shoulders and throwing arm in slingshot fashion toward the direction of throw. (Notice the weight shift and hip action in the javelin throw (see Figure 9.4) and in the golf drive (see Figure 7.4).

"Why should an athlete have his kicking leg extended when contacting the ball in a football punt?"

When the athlete extends the kicking leg, it puts the part of the foot that contacts the ball farther from the kicker's axis of rotation (i.e., the hip joint). Because of this increase in radius, the kicking foot is moving faster than any other part of the leg when it contacts the ball. The flexion of the kicking leg before contact with the ball, together with its extension at impact, simulates a whiplash action (see Figure 9.6).

"Why must an athlete have her center of gravity positioned behind the jumping foot as she enters a high jump takeoff, or behind both feet as she prepares a jump to block or spike in volleyball?"

Positioning the athlete's takeoff foot ahead of the athlete's center of gravity gives the athlete more time to apply force with the jumping leg at takeoff. The athlete rocks forward, up, and then over the jumping foot. This large arc of movement gives the athlete time to drive down at the earth (see Figure 9.3). The earth in reaction drives the athlete upward. The same principle applies to a volleyball spike, a volleyball block, a basketball layup, and a basketball block.

"Why must an athlete extend his body fully at takeoff in a dive that includes multiple somersaults?"

Any time an athlete needs to rotate quickly, the athlete must apply an eccentric or off-center force at takeoff to initiate rotation. The athlete must then pull the body inward from a fully extended position. The large reduction in rotary inertia caused by compacting the body mass around the axis of rotation is rewarded by a huge increase in the rate of spin (i.e., angular velocity) (see Figure 9.9).

"Why must a crawl swimmer use an S-shaped sculling and blading motion with the hands rather than pulling and pushing in a straight line?"

When a crawl swimmer pushes back on the water, the water in reaction pushes the athlete forward. The propulsive force gained from this action is less than the forces that an athlete generates when the hand simulates the blade of a propeller during its S-shaped, downsweep, insweep, and upsweep motion (see Figure 9.2).

"Why should a sprinter's legs and arms thrust and swing parallel to the direction of sprint during a 100 m sprint?"

If a sprinter's arm swing and leg thrust are in any direction other than parallel to the direction of sprint, the forces that the sprinter applies to the earth in the direction of sprint are reduced also. In reaction the force that the earth applies against the sprinter is lessened as well (see Figure 9.1). The result is that the sprinter doesn't run as fast as possible!

Remember all phases and all key elements in a skill are performed for specific mechanical purposes. If you know the mechanical reasons they're performed as they are, you can confidently say to yourself: "O.K. I understand what should occur in the technique of this skill and I understand the mechanical principles behind the movements that the athlete must perform. I'm ready to watch my athlete and I'm ready to correct any errors that I find."

We have asked you to use elite performances as a model when you coach. Don't make the mistake of trying to mold a young athlete in the *exact image* of an elite athlete. What you do when you watch a series of elite performances is to look for, and understand, the *basic technique* that these top athletes use—nothing more. With your knowledge of mechanics you'll see the purpose behind these actions. As you improve as a coach, you'll learn to disregard some actions that a top-class athlete uses because they are personal idiosyncrasies and of no mechanical value. You'd never tell a young athlete that he must hang his tongue out if he wants to shoot as well as Michael Jordan! The same reasoning applies to other elite athletes' personal actions. Accept them as something that makes an individual athlete comfortable, but disregard them as a necessity for good performance.

Remember that actions an elite athlete performs at high velocity over a great range of movement need to be modified to the maturity, strength, flexibility, and endurance of a young athlete. You cannot and must not expect a young, immature athlete, or a novice of any age to assume the body positions or match the explosive actions of an elite athlete. This comes with regular training and good coaching.

SUMMARY

1. Six steps are useful in analyzing a sport skill. The first two steps, "Determine the objectives of the skill" and "Note any special characteristics of the skill," highlight the objectives and conditions governing the performance of a skill. Step 3, "Study top-flight performances of the skill," recommends using performances of elite athletes as models for your coaching. Step 4, "Divide the skill into phases," and Step 5, "Divide each phase into key elements," show the importance of dividing a skill into phases and key elements. Step 6, "Understand the mechanical reasons why a key element is performed as it is," is to understand why the performance of the phases and key elements of a skill must be based on sound mechanical principles.

2. Many skills can be divided into these four phases: preparatory movements and mental set, windup (backswing), force-producing movements, and follow-through (recovery).

3. Key elements are the finer, distinct actions that together make up a phase. Force-producing movements generally contain the most key elements.

REVIEW QUESTIONS

1. The first steps in analyzing a sport skill are to determine the objectives and note any special characteristics of the skill. Why is carrying out these steps important?

2. What is meant by a predictable environment as it relates to the performance of a sport skill? Give two examples of skills normally performed in predictable environments.

3. What must you factor in when you use an elite performance as a model?

4. What is the value of dividing a skill that you are analyzing into phases?

5. What is the purpose of dividing each phase of a skill into its key elements?

6. Why is it important to understand the mechanical reasons for performing each key element in a particular manner?

CHAPTER 8

Identifying and Correcting Errors in Sport Skills

When you finish reading this chapter, you should be able to explain

- how to critically observe the performance of a skill,

- how to analyze each phase of a skill and the key elements within each phase,

- how to make use of knowing sport mechanics in your analysis,

- how to determine the order in which to correct errors, and

- how to select the appropriate coaching methods for correcting errors.

In chapter 7 you went through the first stage in getting ready to correct errors in an athlete's performance. You saw how to break a skill into phases and key elements and understood how the use of sound mechanical principles forms the foundation of good technique. This chapter will give you advice about observing an athlete's performance and using your knowledge of mechanics to pick out errors that need correcting. We have laid out what you must do as a series of five steps:

Step 1. Observe the Complete Skill

Step 2. Analyze Each Phase and Its Key Elements

Step 3. Use Your Knowledge of Sport Mechanics in Your Analysis

Step 4. Select Errors to Be Corrected

Step 5. Decide on Appropriate Methods for the Correction of Errors

Step 1. Observe the Complete Skill

It's a good idea to plan how you intend to observe a skill. By deciding what to look at and where to stand, you can watch the skill or the elements in a phase of the skill as accurately as possible.

Begin by observing (and video recording) your athlete's performance from several different positions. Watch from the left and right, from the front and rear. In this way you can cross-reference and double check the information you gather. Characteristics of the performance that are hidden from one point of view will be revealed

from another. A good approach is to watch the whole skill in this manner several times and then home in on the skill's phases and key elements.

Observing Skills That Contain Distance and Height

Observing skills that contain height and flight, like gymnastic vaults, ski jumping, and pole vault, can be more demanding than skills that contain much less movement, like archery or power lifting. A gymnastic vault contains a long, fast run-up, a takeoff, flight onto and off the horse, and finally a landing. These phases of the skill occur at speed and cover considerable distance and height. To critically observe all aspects of the action, observe from positions that are at right angles and about 15 ft from the flow of the skill. Stand at right angles to the beat-board, then the vaulting horse, and finally position yourself to the rear of the run-up. You can also stand beyond the landing pads so that the athlete runs toward you. In this way you'll get another view of the takeoff, flight, and hand positions on the vaulting box (see Figure 8.1). This observational technique also works well for events in track and field. Figure 8.2

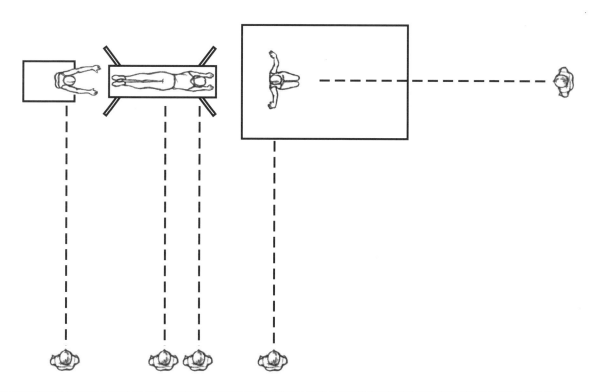

Fig. 8.1. Various viewpoints for assessing a vault in gymnastics.
Adapted from Hay and Reid 1988.

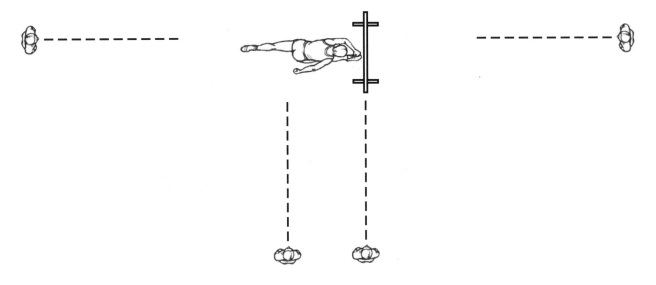

Fig. 8.2. Various viewpoints for assessing a hurdles clearance.

shows a track coach observing from different directions while the athlete practices hurdle clearances. Get closer when skills cover less distance and height and when you are focusing on particular phases and elements of the skill.

Modern television gives us excellent slow-motion coverage of athletes viewed from above. You're probably familiar with the dramatic replays of hand changes on the high bar, swings to a handstand on the rings, and the incredible rotary skills of gymnasts on the pommel horse. In swimming, cameras on tracks on the side and on the bottom of the pool give superb coverage of swimming strokes. If this additional visual information is available, it will help you tremendously with the assessment of your athlete's performance.

Ensuring Safety When Observing

With many skills you'll pick up much worthwhile information when you observe from in front of your athlete. But be particularly careful in this situation. You may center your concentration on your athlete's movements and not on what happens after. Viewing from the front is not recommended with the throwing events in track and field, or with sport skills like golf where the velocity of the ball is exceptional. Unless you have a specially designed protective screen as is used in baseball, be satisfied with viewpoints that are from the side and the rear.

With rotational skills like discus, shot, and hammer, it is best that you are well back behind a safety cage officially approved for the event. This is highly recommended for the discus and hammer throw. In the hammer throw the 16 lb ball travels at phenomenal velocity; in the hands of a novice there is no certainty it will fly in the required direction. If you have no safety cage available, stand well back to the left rear (as you view the athlete from the rear) for hammer and discus throwers who rotate counterclockwise across the ring. In the shot put event (which normally does not use a cage), stand well back to the left rear of right-handed throwers, and vice versa for left-handed throwers. As the athlete becomes a more competent shot-putter, you will be able to move closer without endangering yourself.

If you are assessing your athlete's performance and at the same time marking distances, be aware that an implement in flight is extremely deceptive. Javelins viewed head-on have a habit of momentarily disappearing from sight, and wind can dramatically alter flight paths. Then you must allow for the distances that implements skid and bounce. A discus skidding across wet grass is extremely dangerous!

Finding Settings for Observation

Try to avoid conditions that distract you and your athlete. Physical education classes and recreational settings disturb your concentration and that of your athlete because there are too many other activities going on. If you are instructing a group, you cannot, and should not, pay attention to one athlete for very long. Other athletes need your supervision and encouragement. Any movement in the background can disrupt your attention from the details you want to analyze. The best setting is one in which there are no distractions at all. Your athlete can concentrate on performing and you on observing and analyzing.

Getting Started With Your Observation

Have your athlete warm up and perform the skill several times so you get a good overall impression. Don't concentrate on specific phases, even though a poor windup or a poor force-producing phase will obviously catch your eye. Try to get a feel for your athlete's rhythm, flow, and general body positions from the start of the skill to the finish. Your main objective at this stage is to get an overall impression of your athlete's performance.

Giving Comments During Observation

When you observe, don't distract your athlete by continuously offering instruction. Watch without making any comments other than an occasional encouraging remark after the skill is completed. Try to keep your athlete relaxed and enjoying the situation of having you as an enthusiastic and knowledgeable spectator. Your athlete should not struggle to impress you, be discouraged, or become so casual that she loses concentration. You want an accurate impression of your athlete's abilities, not a performance altered by tension or insufficient concentration. Above all, don't start listing aloud all the actions your athlete is doing wrong! This serves no purpose and destroys your athlete's morale. You don't want your athlete to become tense or stressed in any way. Your job is to get a true impression of how your athlete performs.

While you observe, make a mental note if you think your athlete is lacking in strength, flexibility, or endurance. Your athlete cannot change these characteristics during one training session just as she cannot gain or lose weight on command. Take these factors into account by modifying your demands when you start correcting errors. In other training sessions you can get your athlete to work for improvement in these areas.

Observing Skills Performed at Normal Speed

When you observe the complete skill for the first time, it is best if your athlete performs the skill at normal speed. The reason for this recommendation is that skills performed at unnaturally slow speeds are dramatically different from those that occur at normal speed. Timing, coordination, and the feel for the skill are different. Slow speed performances serve little purpose when you are looking for errors to correct. They give you a false picture of what is occurring. Reduce speed when you teach some new pattern of movements. When the fundamentals are learned, the speed of movement can be increased.

Determining the Number of Times You Observe a Skill

How often you watch your athlete perform depends on the physical demands of the skill. Skills that take considerable time, concentration, and effort for each repetition, such as diving and ski jumping, are by necessity viewed fewer times than a place kick, a volleyball serve, a pass in soccer, or the repetitive paddling actions of a kayaker. It is important however, that you view the performance enough times so your athlete's pattern of movements becomes apparent. With skills like diving and ski jumping you may need to use more than one training session to develop an accurate impression of your athlete's abilities.

Differences Between Beginners and Experienced Athletes

As you observe, expect that a beginner's performance will change dramatically from one repetition of the skill to the next, and that the beginner will tire more quickly than an experienced athlete. Novices make gross errors in which they miss several key elements in a phase, or even a whole phase of a skill. During your general observation you'll notice that their foot positions are incorrect at one moment and correct the next. You'll notice that the beginner does not use the large muscles of the body, and does not shift the body weight in the correct direction. You may even feel, after completing the observation, that the best course of action is to totally rebuild the skill. With novices you must accept this situation. It's part of coaching beginners!

In comparison to beginners you'll find that experienced athletes make fewer apparent errors. You'll easily see these errors when you analyze a slow-motion video of the skill, or you'll catch them when you concentrate on specific elements in the skill. Perhaps you'll discover that your athlete's line of vision is incorrect, or that the head is in the wrong position, upsetting the athlete's balance. You may discover that your athlete's overall performance is good except that the wrist action at the end of a pitch, throw, or hit is not as it should be. You may have to struggle through many training sessions to get an experienced athlete to eliminate these seemingly minor errors. The reason for this difficulty is that an elite athlete has probably ground in the incorrect action and has been performing it this way for years. How different it is when you coach a young novice! Every coaching session can be a giant leap forward! To your delight you'll find that the technique of most young novices is like clay that you can mold. Each coaching session can make a massive change in the quality of their performance. This is why many coaches find great pleasure in coaching young novices!

Observing and Spotting

If you are a novice coach, you may find it difficult to critically observe a performance when you are also involved in spotting. Your attention tends to be on where you should give support (and perhaps protecting yourself from the flailing arms and legs!), rather than judging whether certain movements are performed correctly. In gymnastics, dividing your attention can be a risky practice. Experienced coaches can carry out both jobs at once, but even these coaches have to concentrate on their spotting when more exotic skills are attempted. If you are starting as a coach in a sport that has a high level of risk, play it safe and use competent spotters if you want to be free to observe. If spotters are not available, have an onlooker videotape the performer while you give the necessary assistance. Afterward analyze and discuss the performance with the athlete.

Looking for Other Clues

Part of your observation technique will be to look beyond your athlete for clues about the perfor-

mance. The flight path, rebound, and roll of balls result from the movements and actions your athlete uses in the skill. Skate marks on ice, ski patterns on snow, footprints on run-ups, takeoffs, and landings are all clues to what's going on in the skill.

Don't forget to use your ears as well as your eyes when you look for clues! The rhythm of footfalls during a run-up or during the repetitive bounding of a triple jump is an indication of stride length and stride cadence. The overemphasized thud of one of your athlete's feet during throwing events is a sure sign of poor balance and weight distribution. (It's also a sure sign that the hop or the step in the triple jump is too large!) The noise of bat and club on ball are clues to a direct or sliced impact. In volleyball, a slapping noise is a giveaway to the coach of a carried ball or some other incorrect contact. Almost every sport will give you visual and auditory signals that you'll be able to associate with good or bad performance. Use every source of information. Don't limit yourself in any way.

Step 2. Analyze Each Phase and Its Key Elements

After you have watched the complete skill several times, you are ready to concentrate on individual phases and their key elements. There are two ways to approach this.

Start With the Result

One method coaches commonly use with an athlete who is competent is to start with the end product and work back from there. Here's an example: A punter is trying to spiral a football for distance. There's enough force put into the kick but there's no spiral. So you concentrate on the action of the foot as it contacts the ball. Is the ball fed onto the kicker's foot correctly? Is the kicker's foot drawn across the long axis of the ball to produce the torque necessary to spiral the ball? On the other hand, if the ball's spiral is satisfactory but distance is lacking, then shift your attention to other phases and key elements in the skill. Ask yourself, "Is there an adequate shift of the kicker's body into the kick?" "Are the lower leg and kicking foot allowed to swing freely or is the kicker tightening the leg muscles and eliminating any chance of a whiplash action occurring?" "Is flexibility a problem?" If it is, then it will restrict the range that the kicking leg swings through and reduce the force applied to the ball.

In throwing, kicking, and striking skills, checking the result gives you a wealth of information. You might have a big, powerful athlete who ought to throw the shot a long distance, but there's no force behind the shot and you know the athlete should be throwing 10 ft farther. So you concentrate on the throwing stance that the athlete assumes after the glide across the ring is complete. When you examine the throwing stance, you ask yourself, "Is the athlete's body angled correctly?" "Are the shoulders still facing the rear of the ring when the glide is complete?" "Is the foot placement correct?" "Is the athlete rotating the hips toward the direction of throw, and are the massive muscles of the legs, seat, and back used before the chest, arm, and fingers?" (Figure 8.3 shows the actions that you should be looking for in shot put!) After critically examining the throwing stance, you may decide that the problem lies in a poor glide across the ring. Well-performed standing throws confirm your suspicion. The athlete's glide across the ring is ruining the remaining part of the throw! You and your athlete get to work to correct the errors in this phase of the throw.

Observe Each Phase of the Skill in Sequence

Another method of observation that coaches commonly use is to start by critically observing the first phase in the skill, then progress to the second, third, and so on. The first phase contains preliminary movements and your athlete's establishment of a mental set. Then you shift your attention to the second phase, which will be the windup.

In the first phase you'll look at such elements as your athlete's stance and weight distribution. You'll take note of your athlete's head position, line of vision, and the way your athlete concentrates for the actions that will follow. When your athlete winds up, or performs a backswing, you'll examine your athlete's weight transference from one foot to the other. (Figure 7.4 a-b illustrates the athlete's body position, weight shift, and backswing in a golf drive.) You'll check the position of the implement and your athlete's body at the end

of the windup. Make a mental note if your athlete appears stiff and needs to improve flexibility.

When you examine the force-producing phase, remember that in many skills this phase is made up of several distinct sections, such as a run-up and a takeoff in jumps and vaults, a run-up, glide, spin, and throw in throwing events, or an approach, hurdle step, board flexion, and takeoff in springboard dives. In front crawl, it can be the "catch" of the water at hand entry followed by the outsweep, insweep, downsweep, and upsweep motion of the swimmer's hand. Break these complicated force-producing phases into key elements and concentrate on each key element in sequence.

In most skills the follow-through is the least important of all phases. Your athlete has applied force and the follow-through safely dissipates the athlete's momentum and kinetic energy. But be sure to observe what happens during the follow-through and, of course, what happens to the implement and your athlete immediately afterward! Your athlete's actions and the implement's flight are clues to what has happened earlier. Check your athlete's arm and hand actions during the follow-through on a jump shot in basketball or a volleyball spike. In these skills, a follow-through can indicate the amount and direction of force and spin that's applied to the ball.

In some sport skills, insufficient control during the force-producing phase produces a follow-through that causes a violation of the rules of the sport. A field hockey player swings the stick too high, and the volleyball player hits the net after spiking or blocking. Don't disregard the follow-through, but look on it as an important phase that will give you clues to what happened during the windup and force-producing phases that occurred earlier.

In cyclic, repetitive skills like swimming, remember that the follow-through is a recovery action that sets your athlete up for another force-producing phase. Check that these recovery actions are mechanically efficient and not wasting your athlete's energy. A misdirected arm recovery in the crawl, in which the swimmer's arm swings across the midline of the body, produces poor body alignment, generates excessive form drag, and affects the efficiency of the force-producing phase that follows (see Figure 8.4). Cyclists talk of the need to spin the pedals meaning that proper pedaling technique is a rotary motion, not just a push downward with a rest on the way up. Check that your athlete is pulling up

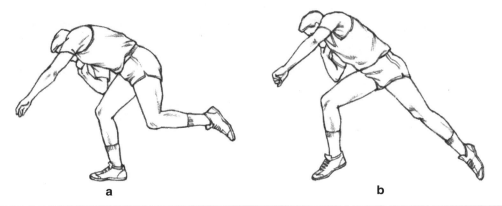

Fig. 8.3. Excellent technique in the shot put.

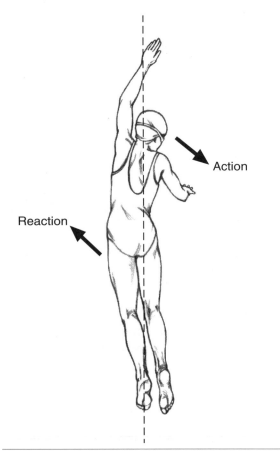

Action

Reaction

Fig. 8.4. Overreaching and crossing the midline with an arm entry causes the hips to react and move in the opposing direction.
Adapted from Maglischo 1983.

and around with one leg while pushing down and around with the other. Proper pedaling technique is the ultimate in cyclic repetitive action.

Step 3. Use Your Knowledge of Sport Mechanics in Your Analysis

As you observe each successive phase and its key elements (from preliminary movements and mental set to follow-through or recovery), you must put your knowledge of sport mechanics to work. **In particular, concentrate on how your athlete applies muscular force to produce a desired action in a skill.** You must carefully assess the mechanical efficiency of your athlete's actions and the way your athlete competes against gravity, friction, drag, air resistance, the forces generated by opponents, or whatever the opposition is! In this way you can pick out technical (i.e., mechanical) errors that your athlete commits. What should you be looking for as you examine the elements in each phase? Here is a series of important questions you can ask yourself as a guide.

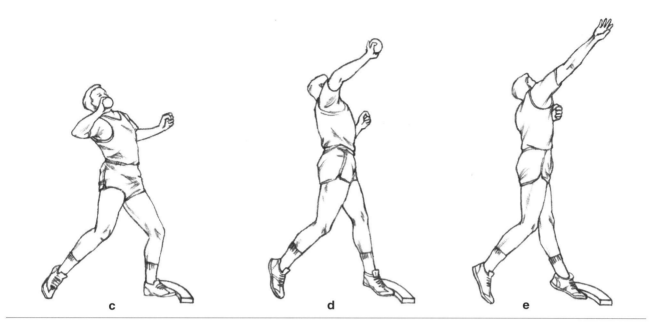

c   d   e

• **Does your athlete have optimal stability when applying or receiving force?** A wide base and correctly positioned center of gravity are essential for applying and receiving force. Check the position of your athlete's center of gravity and the way your athlete sets up a base of support. Ask yourself the following questions:

"Is my athlete's base of support extended in the direction it should be?"

"Is the base too narrow or too wide?"

"Is my athlete standing too erect instead of squatting down?"

"Is my athlete's center of gravity too close to the edge of the base when it should be centralized?"

If your athlete stumbles or gets thrown one way as the implement goes the other, or if your athlete is too easily knocked off balance by an opponent, you'll know there's an error in this area. So check through the mechanical principles associated with balance, equilibrium, and stability. Remember that stability is one turning effect (i.e., torque) battling another, and to remain stable your athlete may have to reposition her feet and center of gravity to apply more leverage and more torque.

In many skills, your athlete wants to be able to move quickly and to react in an instant! When your athlete is receiving a serve, playing in goal,

or reacting to the moves of an opponent, maximum stability is not the objective, but rather a level of stability that allows your athlete to move in a flash in any direction! We discussed these principles in detail in chapter 5.

In particular be sure that you carefully check the size and alignment of your athlete's base of support and the position of her center of gravity during a skill's force-producing phase. An inadequate base not only makes your athlete unstable but, equally important, it reduces the distance and time over which your athlete can apply force.

• **Is your athlete using all the muscles that can make a contribution to the skill?** Athletes produce inferior performances because they do not apply force with all the muscles they can and should use in a skill. This may seem a strange state of affairs! After all, why not use the muscles of the legs, or in any other part of the body if these muscles can make a contribution to the performance? If the performance of a skill requires the muscles of the legs, trunk, chest, and arms, and your athlete uses only the muscles of the chest and arms, then the total force put into the skill will be below optimal level. How can you tell if your athlete is using the muscles? Usually this is easy because in dynamic skills muscle contractions produce actions! If a limb segment or some other part of the body moves, you know muscles are contracting. Here's an example of what we mean. When you watch a child throw a ball for distance for the first time, you'll notice that the youngster frequently stands still with the feet close together, then throws with the arm alone. There's no wide throwing stance. The throwing arm is not taken back, nor are the shoulders rotated away from the direction of throw. In the force-producing phase of the throw, the muscles in the legs make no contribution, nor do the muscles surrounding the trunk and chest. This error doesn't only occur among children. You'll see it happening among adults as well.

Top-flight athletes always aim to have all the required muscle groups contributing to the skill. Elite rowers make sure that the muscles of the legs, back, shoulders, and arms play their part in the stroke. Speed skaters like Bonnie Blair and Dan Jansen make sure that their leg muscles contribute optimally in powering them along the ice. The muscles working their arms and shoulders make their own contribution in counterbalancing the actions of the legs. Imagine how poor Bonnie's performance would be if she failed to use her quadriceps muscles adequately to extend the legs, or if she skated with the arms hanging straight down instead of forcefully swinging them back and forth! The same principle applies to all skills. Make sure that all members of your athlete's muscular team are making a contribution by moving the body segments that they are responsible for moving! Think of your athlete's muscles as members of a tug-of-war team. If a team is made of eight members, why have one or more of the team resting on the rope without pulling?

• **Is your athlete applying force with the muscles in the correct sequence?** If a world champion weight lifter like Karyn Marshall performs a clean and jerk, and you critically examine the key elements of her clean (in which she pulls the bar up to her chest), you'll see that Karyn contracts the muscles of her legs, back, shoulders, and arms at about the same time. The extension of Karyn's legs is closely linked to an extension of her back and a strong upward pull with her arms. On the other hand, if you examine the key elements in the force-producing phase of a pitcher's fastball, you'll see a well-defined sequence of actions, starting from the big muscles that accelerate the athlete's body and the athlete's large, more massive body segments, and finishing with the high-speed movement of smaller, less massive body segments (i.e., the throwing arm and hand, with

the baseball). All great pitchers step forward as the throwing arm is drawn back and the shoulders are rotated away from the batter. When they have stepped out into the pitching stance, their bodies rotate toward the hitter in a whiplike sequence that starts from the legs, shifts to the hips, then to the chest, and ends with a tremendous acceleration of the throwing arm. The pitcher's body acts like the handle of a whip that is being cracked. The hand gripping the baseball is the tip of the whip! A spike in volleyball by Karch Kiraly, or a serve in tennis by Steffi Graf use a similar whiplike sequence of actions.

A comparison between the actions used in a clean and jerk and a baseball pitch demonstrates opposite extremes in the sequence that an athlete's muscle contractions occur. When you examine each phase in your athlete's performance, check that the movement of your athlete's limb segments occurs in the correct sequence. If they do, then you know that muscle contractions are occurring in the correct sequence as well. A common fault for many athletes in throwing and hitting skills is to use the small muscles of the shoulders and throwing arm long before the big muscles of the legs, back, and trunk have done their job. The result is that the big muscles never get the heavier parts of the body moving ahead of those that are lighter. It's impossible to crack a whip if you don't accelerate the whip handle first!

• **Is your athlete applying the right amount of muscular force over the appropriate time frame?** You'll recognize this statement as our old friend "impulse," which we discussed in chapter 3. Remember that impulse refers not only to the amount of force that your athlete uses, but also to the time period that your athlete applies force.

If your athlete uses the right amount of force for the right amount of time, your athlete's limbs move at the required speed through the required range of movement. When this occurs and all muscle contractions are sequenced correctly, you'll see movements that are fluid, smooth, rhythmic, graceful, and well coordinated. When an athlete applies force indiscriminately and haphazardly (and this is what novices do!), you'll see actions that are jerky and awkward. What you are seeing is the difference between a polished and well-practiced technique, and one that is not!

Practice helps your athlete establish how much force each muscle involved in a skill must exert. When they are learning, many athletes apply too much or too little force at the wrong time and, as a result, their technique will look jerky and awkward. You can help your athlete correct this situation by giving rhythmic cues that provide an idea of the speed at which the athlete should perform the actions. You can also provide coaching tips like, "Step out long and low, and as soon as your foot hits the deck, thrust your hips toward the direction you are throwing" or "Stretch up at takeoff and swing your arms upward as fast as you can!"

Keep in mind that what is correct in a mechanical sense is not always possible in an anatomical sense. In other words, mechanical principles must fit with the design of your athlete's body. For example, athletes *do not* apply maximum force over the *longest* possible time frame even in hitting skills that require maximum velocity at impact, or in jumping skills that require maximum velocity at takeoff. In these skills, good technique is characterized by limbs that are slightly flexed at the start of the skill and fully extended from maximal muscular contraction when impact and takeoff occur. Look for this action when you examine the final elements of the force-producing phases in golf, baseball batting, tennis serving, and track and field throwing.

In skills that require accuracy, like a volley in tennis or a drop shot in squash, look for controlled force applied over a specific range. Too much force or too great a range of movement defeats the purpose of the skill. When too much force or too great a range of movement occurs, the volley puts the ball out of the court. Likewise a drop shot in squash rebounds too high from the front wall making the "get" easy for the opponent.

A word of advice in relation to force and the time frame that force is applied. No one expects young novices to be able to produce the same force as adults, and likewise, you cannot expect novices to assume the same body positions and apply force over the time frame and distances elite athletes use. Make allowances when you watch your young athlete perform. Less force applied over a limited range of movement is not necessarily an error but a stage in the developmental process. More force and a greater range of movement will come with increased strength, flexibility, endurance, and coordination—all of which are carefully molded by your good coaching.

• **Is your athlete applying force in the correct direction?** This principle may seem to you hardly worth mentioning, yet you should look for this factor, particularly in the force-producing phase of the skill. Sprinters like Michael Johnson, Carl Lewis, and Gwen Torrence drive down and back with each leg thrust so they travel forward at the greatest possible velocity toward the finishing line. The direction of each leg thrust gives these superb athletes the exact amount of vertical and horizontal thrust required by each sprinting stride. The result is optimal forward propulsion. You'd have no trouble deciding that there was something terribly wrong with Gwen's technique if her leg thrust was directed out to the side, or if

Franz Klammer Combined Innovative Technique With Super Coaching and Equipment

At the 1976 Winter Games in Innsbruck, downhill skier Franz Klammer thrilled the world with his hair-raising gold medal performance. Franz's rocketing do-or-die performance is still considered one of the most exciting and brilliant downhill runs in the history of modern ski racing. In remembering that run 20 years ago, Franz said he was helped immensely by superior coaching and equipment. He also said that a large part of his success came from an innovative way in which he carved his turns. At that time, ski racers used to skid through their turns on the flats of their skis. Franz started his turn with the ski on its edge. With less skidding at the beginning of the turn, Franz came out of his turns with more speed than his rivals. Since Innsbruck, in a World Cup career that has spanned nearly 15 years, Franz has amassed 25 downhill victories, the most of any downhill ski racer. In 1975 and 1976 he won 13 World Cup downhills in a row, a record that remains unbroken.

her arms swung sideways across her body rather than forward and backward! Errors like these in the force-producing phase of sprinting indicate that the athlete is wasting force and not applying it in the correct direction.

In your analysis of the performance of sport skills, you'll notice that inexperienced athletes apply force in many different directions. They waste much of their muscular effort so it makes no contribution to their performance. Look also for inexperienced athletes to thrust and push in the correct direction with one part of their bodies, and in an incorrect direction with another part. Their torsos go one way and their throwing or hitting arms go another! Young shot-putters often complain that the shot bends their fingers backward. A careful examination of the arm action in their throws indicates that they are not pushing directly behind the center of gravity of the shot. The thrust is in some other direction and the result is that the shot bends their fingers back. Likewise, a hammer thrower or discus thrower who spins on the spot instead of traveling across the ring, or who falls sideways out of the ring when he releases the implement, is obviously misdirecting his force! Poorly directed force produces inadequate rotation at takeoff for gymnasts, divers, and skaters; mishits in sports that use clubs, bats, and racquets; miskicks in sports that use kicking skills; and poor propulsion in swimming skills.

• **Is your athlete correctly applying torque and momentum transfer?** Many sport skills require your athlete to generate and control rotation. Rotation is applied to your athlete's body, an opponent, a ball, or an implement like a discus. To initiate rotation your athlete must apply the turning effect of torque. The more spin required, the more torque your athlete has to apply. In your analysis, check how much force your athlete is generating and the distance this force is applied relative to the axis of rotation. For your athlete to apply more spiral to a football, he must grip around the middle, fatter portion of the ball. More torque is applied in this manner. In judo, look at the position of the axis of rotation that your athlete sets up for a hip throw and where your athlete applies force to the opponent. Is your athlete strong enough to apply tremendous force? If not, is there any way of increasing the force arm (i.e., the distance from the axis to where force is applied)? The larger this distance the less effort your athlete must apply.

In gymnastics, diving, and figure skating the number of rotations your athlete performs de-

pends on how much torque your athlete generates and how much momentum transfer your athlete uses at takeoff. Momentum comes largely from arm and leg actions that are transferred at takeoff to your athlete's body as a whole. Check the actions of the arms and the free leg to see whether they make an adequate contribution to your athlete's rotation. A skater who performs a double spin when intending to perform a triple may say, "I don't think I got enough spin!" After you've analyzed the skater's takeoff you may disagree! You might decide that sufficient torque was applied at takeoff, and in fact it was overemphasized! Your analysis may indicate instead that there was not enough upward thrust at takeoff and that the arms and free leg were not swung vigorously enough to provide any transfer of momentum in an upward direction to the skater's body.

• **Is your athlete decreasing rotary resistance to spin faster and increasing rotary resistance to spin slower?** If a skill requires your athlete to spin faster, turn quicker, or swing the limbs at high speed, your athlete must decrease her rotary resistance (i.e., rotary inertia) by pulling her body in toward her axis of rotation. The requirements of the skill determine the tightness of this position. Arms flexed at the elbows help to produce a fast and efficient arm swing for sprinters and speed skaters. A tight tuck for gymnasts and a compressed body position for skaters when they spin around their long axis helps to produce the required number of rotations. Extended body positions oppose a fast spin and slow down rotation. Is your athlete not tucking tight enough because of insufficient flexibility or lack of muscular strength, or is the problem inadequate knowledge of the correct timing in the skill? Your careful analysis of each phase and its key elements can pinpoint the source of the problem.

Keep in mind that when your athlete rotates and extends the arms, her body slows, but her arms and hands travel faster. Put a racquet or a bat in your athlete's hand and the head of the implement travels fastest of all. Many skills require a combination of hip and shoulder rotation coupled with full extension of the arm (particularly at impact or release). For example, a tennis player and a golfer must have full arm extension when the racquet or club hits the ball. A discus thrower must release the discus with the implement as far from the body as possible. In your analysis, look for extension at release and impact, and for some flexion and tighter body positions earlier in the skill.

Step 4. Select Errors to Be Corrected

After you've analyzed each phase and its key elements, you have the task of deciding the sequence that you'll follow in correcting errors. Like any enthusiastic coach you'd like to correct every error in the first training session. The difficulty you'll face is that inexperienced athletes commit numerous errors, some of which are major and some minor. What is a major error and what is a minor error?

A major error will be the absence or poor performance of any item that we've discussed under Step 3 in this chapter. So, errors that destroy your athlete's stability or the optimal use of your athlete's muscular force are major errors. A minor error is an action that only partially detracts from the performance of the skill. Examples of minor errors are a backswing in golf that needs to travel a few degrees farther back, a throwing stance that needs to extend a little farther, an arm swing at takeoff in a jumping event that needs to be more vigorous. To an elite athlete, minor errors of this nature make the difference between a good performance and a world record. To a coach working with a beginner they are errors that can be placed on the back burner while other more important errors are corrected.

The simple method to follow in selecting errors is to forget those that are minor and pick out those that are major. When you've picked out the major errors, select the one that has the most adverse effect on the skill and work on this error first. If you still have trouble deciding which error to choose, home in on major errors in your athlete's stance and body position—particularly in the preliminary stance and in the force-producing phase. Get the preliminary stance straightened out and then shift to the force-producing phase. Why? Because an athlete cannot apply force correctly unless stance and body position are correct. In throwing, hitting and striking skills, and in contact sports, poor position and lack of balance destroy everything! An incorrect stance will ruin a golf stroke, and an incorrect body position simply sets a wrestler up for a countermove. In swimming, a body position where the athlete is not horizontal in the water creates tremendous form drag. Keeping the head down and improving the leg kick can correct this. It's amazing how much faster a swimmer will travel when a drooping body is raised into a horizontal position!

Step 5. Decide on Appropriate Methods for the Correction of Errors

This step leads you from sport mechanics into methods of teaching and coaching sport skills. Errors in skill performances vary in complexity. At their most complex, errors can be mistimed sequences of high-speed arm actions occurring in flight as a diver combines a somersault with a twist. At their simplest, a young novice might have the wrong leg forward when throwing a softball. If you are coaching the diver, you have the options of discussion, video analysis, and demonstration of the correct arm actions from the side of the pool. If you are lucky enough to coach at a pool with high-tech equipment, with a press of a button you can foam up the water with air bubbles so your diver can work on the arm actions knowing that she's not going to get hurt if she fails! You might also decide that the correct arm actions need to be reinforced over and over on the trampoline with your diver in a spotting belt. But once your diver is in flight there's no possibility of hands-on help from you, and your athlete has no chance of slowing the skill in any way. It's the same when you coach a basketball layup or a start in swimming. It's obviously easier when you teach a youngster to throw a softball. You can demonstrate and say, "Put your left leg forward and turn your right shoulder to the rear as you take your arm back!" You can even move the youngster's limbs into the correct position. It's impossible to do this with a diver in flight or a swimmer leaving the blocks!

Because sport skills vary so much and errors are so diverse, it's impossible to offer you a single method that works for the correction of all errors. What we have listed below is a step-by-step sequence that will help in most situations you'll encounter.

Steps in Error Correction

- If possible, separate the phase that contains the error from the rest of the skill. Treat this phase and its key elements as a skill in itself.

- Break the phase and its elements into smaller parts. For example, if the error is poor synchronization of footwork and arm actions, consider teaching the footwork first. Then teach the arm actions. Later add the two together. Use verbal counts and rhythmic cues to assist your athlete.

- Choose an activity that is useful for teaching the correct movements. Activities should be easy to perform and if possible novel and interesting to the performer. Above all, be creative and flexible in your approach. If the activity you choose doesn't help to correct the error, don't be afraid to change it. What will work well for one of your athletes may not work so well for another.

- Whenever possible have your athlete perform new movements slowly.

- Walk your athlete through the required body positions, pausing wherever appropriate. Again use a verbal count for rhythm.

- Increase the speed of performance slowly. Always be prepared to repeat a step in this progression if speed reintroduces errors.

- When you have decided that the actions you wanted to correct are learned well enough, put them back into the phase they came from, and check your athlete's performance. If you are satisfied, attach additional phases from the skill at either end of the one containing the correction. Check how your athlete integrates the new movements. If problems persist, reinforce earlier steps in this sequence.

- Attempt the complete skill at reduced speed and effort with the corrected movements in place.

- Progressively increase speed and effort.

Safety in Coaching High Risk Skills

As we mentioned earlier, in many skills it's impossible for the athlete to pause halfway through and rethink movements! These skills usually involve flight and often have a high element of risk. A back somersault in gymnastic floor exercises is such a skill. With skills of this nature we recommend the following sequence:

- Maximize safety with spotters, overhead spotting rigs, safety belts, crash pads, pits filled with foam rubber, or any other specialized equipment that fully protects the performer. In this way your athlete can perform the required actions with confidence and without danger.

- With highly complex skills, go back to a known skill that contains elements of the movement patterns you wish to correct. Use this skill to reinforce the correct actions.

A Coach's Responsibility

For many female gymnasts, the toughest piece of equipment they have to face is not the beam or the uneven bars, but the scale where they must constantly monitor their body weight. Some female gymnasts have been told that they are too fat to win at 100 lb and because of the pressure have suffered from bulimia and anorexia. Competing at a high level, young female gymnasts are well aware of the importance of a superior strength to weight ratio, and equally important, that gymnastics, like synchronized swimming, figure skating, and diving, is an aesthetic sport where looks count! Male gymnasts suffer less from bulimia and anorexia, but the problem exists in sports like wrestling, boxing, and judo where making the weight is essential. As a coach, it is important that you understand how talent, training, technique, and determination combine to produce a superior performance. At the same time you must not forget that you have a responsibility for your athlete's well-being. Winning is great, but a well-adjusted and happy athlete after a sport career is over is more important!

- Progressively remove spotters and other specialized equipment as the skill is learned.
- When your athlete attempts the skill alone, provide experienced spotting that can provide assistance if it's necessary.

Your Attitude During the Correction Process

During whatever process of correcting errors you use, remain positive and praise good effort and correct performance. Your objective is to have your athlete persevere through those difficult periods when she feels that the correct action will never be mastered. The progress your athlete makes will depend on the amount of practice, the complexity of the required actions, and how long it takes you and your athlete to mold the corrected action into the total skill.

Giving Advice to Your Athlete

How you and your athlete communicate determines how much success you gain when you attempt to correct errors. Don't befuddle a young athlete with needless technical jargon. Translate your mechanical know-how into instructions that fit the age, intelligence, and physical ability of your athlete. Some athletes will be genuinely interested in the mechanical principles behind a movement. Statements like, "Straighten your arms when you contact the ball—it'll help you to apply more force" are excellent because they indicate in easy to understand language the mechanical reasons behind a body position. But for most athletes, comments about angular momentum, momentum transfer, kinetic energy, and rotary inertia are meaningless! For most athletes, the less cluttered their minds, the freer they are to perform. This recommendation also relates to the amount of information you give at any one time in your instructions. Give simple, short, easy to understand instructions that are to the point. No athlete wants to stand around while the coach talks endlessly about what could or should be done.

Improving Feedback

Few sports use mirrors the way that bodybuilders do. Besides providing the bodybuilders with continuous aesthetic assessment, mirrors provide instant visual feedback on how they perform an exercise. In the highly dynamic actions of most sports, the nearest you can get to a mirrored image is an immediate playback on a video machine. The machine tells your athlete, "This is what you looked like." Neither the machine nor a mirror can say, "This is what the movements should feel like." Your athlete is the only one who actually feels the movement. As a coach observing and assessing the skill you cannot feel what your athlete feels although you can say to your athlete, "It should feel like this." To be able to provide this kind of information requires considerable experience from you, first as an athlete and then as a coach.

Sometimes you'll be surprised at the response when you ask, "What did you feel at that moment in the skill?" Many novices have no idea what happened, and they have no sense of where their limbs are as they attempt a skill. Elite athletes differ considerably. Most of them have a well-developed kinesthetic sense and are aware of what their bodies are doing during a performance. Teach young athletes to develop this sensory awareness. It becomes an invaluable resource in helping them to master sport skills.

Consider the Time Available for Correcting Errors

One factor that will have considerable influence on you will be the time that you have available to work with your athlete. Can you plan a training program that stretches over several months or a year, or are you working with a 3- to 6-week block before the competitive season starts? When you are restricted by time, it affects your choice of errors and the methods you use to correct them. You may feel that all you can do is correct some minor errors, because major changes initially make your athlete perform poorly and this downtime can carry into the competitive season. Whenever an athlete has to think what he is doing in one or more phases of a skill, the effect is a drop in performance. The correct action has to become second nature—an unconscious action. Remember that correcting a minor error can have a considerable effect on performance. Be satisfied with that! Save large changes in technique for the off-season.

Getting Additional Help

You have to gather information from many different sources if you want to become a good coach in your chosen sport. In the area of analysis and correction of skills, you should be ready to do the following:

- Read texts on your sport that offer successful teaching methods and techniques for correcting errors. The best texts should offer excellent illustrations of lead-ups and teaching progressions. A quality text contains lists of the common errors that occur in the skills of your sport, with explanations on how to correct them. Look also for safety recommendations, not only for individuals, but also for group activities. This is particularly important when you are teaching skills that have a high element of risk.

- Plan to attend coaching seminars and workshops. Here you can listen to presentations on coaching from experienced coaches and experts who do research in your area. You can discuss problems in your sport with coaches who are aware of the latest coaching techniques. Join your local and national coaching association so you can regularly receive the latest newsletters.

- Modern video and computer technology now give you the opportunity to analyze performances in superslow motion and to place elite performances on the same screen as those of novices. This is of tremendous assistance when you want to look at differences in technique. Computer advances in virtual reality now offer you and your athlete a "virtually real" method of experiencing the movement patterns of a skill while remaining static. Previously downhill skiers and luge competitors would close their eyes and imagine steering through the curves and straightaways. With virtual reality your athlete can put on a specially designed helmet that feeds a 3-D image containing an accurate representation of the bends, twists, and straightaways that exist on the course. A computer will have worked out the best course to follow relative to ice temperatures and other weather conditions. This remarkable computer simulation was used in preparation for the 1994 Winter Olympic Games in Lillehammer, Norway.

- Read beyond this book and improve your knowledge of mechanics as it applies to your sport. Don't become tunnel-visioned—take an interest in other sports as well! It will make you more of an expert in your own!

SUMMARY

1. There are five steps to the effective observation, analysis, and correction of errors in sport skills. These are to (1) observe the complete skill, (2) analyze each phase and its key elements, (3) use your knowledge of sport mechanics in making an analysis, (4) select errors to be corrected, and (5) decide on appropriate coaching techniques for the correction of errors.

2. Observe skills from several different positions; avoid settings in which you and your athlete are distracted. Use video recordings to assist in your analysis.

3. Do not concentrate on skill analysis while you are providing safety or involved in spotting the performer.

4. Once you have a good overall impression of an athletic performance, analyze each successive phase of the skill together with its key elements.

5. Use your knowledge of sport mechanics for analyzing performance. Ask yourself mechanical questions (e.g., Does the athlete have maximum stability when applying or receiving force?).

6. Divide the performance errors you see into major and minor categories. Major errors seriously detract from the optimal performance of the skill, whereas minor errors have minimal effect on performance. Follow the sequence outlined in this chapter for correcting errors.

7. Use the very best safety techniques when correcting errors in skills that contain a high level of risk.

8. Maintain a positive attitude during the correction process. Avoid using technical jargon excessively during coaching sessions.

9. Teach athletes to develop sensory awareness to assist them in error correction.

10. Be aware of the time you have available for correcting errors. Do not attempt massive changes in technique if time is limited.

11. Attend coaching seminars and read texts on your sport that offer top quality teaching methods and techniques for the correction of errors. Be alert to any advances in computer and video technology that can assist you in coaching. Expand your knowledge of sport mechanics, not only in your sport but in other sports as well.

REVIEW QUESTIONS

1. What is a good sequence to follow in analyzing each phase of a sport skill?

2. What is the mechanical difference between the recovery in a swimming stroke and the follow-through in a throwing skill ?

3. What is the common appearance of a skill when an athlete tries to use more than the optimal number of muscles in a performance? Give a common example of an athlete applying muscular force in the wrong sequence to perform a skill.

4. Why is it important for an athlete to apply the right amount of force over the appropriate time frame with each of the muscles involved in a sport skill?

5. What does this text refer to as major errors in the performance of a skill?

6. What resources can you use to assist you in becoming a better coach in your sport?

CHAPTER 9

Mechanics of Selected Sport Skills

In this chapter we analyze a number of sport skills to show you how technique and mechanics are inseparable. As you read the following pages, you'll find that they are a good review of the mechanical principles you've read about earlier in this book.

We describe the technique and mechanics of 11 sport skills on the following pages. Under "technique," you'll find the skill's most important technical characteristics. Technique tells you what should occur when athletes sprint, swim the front crawl, high jump, and so forth. Under "mechanics," you'll find a description of mechanical principles at work during the technique.

This is where you'll find the mechanical reasons a skill is performed the way it is! In this way you can immediately read the mechanical reasons behind each phase of a skill an athlete performs.

This analysis does not cover every sport skill that exists, nor satisfy the needs of every coach. But we've tried to cover a wide range of sports. If this review highlights for you how technique and mechanics are intrinsically tied together, and how you cannot teach technique without knowing mechanics, then it's done its job!

Table 9.1 lists the sport skills you'll find in this appendix and our rationale for including them.

Table 9.1 Sport Skills

General skill	Specific skill	Rationale
Running	Sprinting	All athletes use sprinting as a form of locomotion. It is the most dynamic and vigorous of all running techniques. Walking and middle- and long-distance running obey the same mechanical laws as sprinting but use less vigorous actions.
Swimming	Front crawl	The front crawl is the most popular and fastest of all major swimming strokes. The mechanical principles that govern the technique used in the front crawl apply to other swimming strokes as well as to the sculling actions used in water polo and synchronized swimming.
Jumping	High jump	The mechanical principles that control how an athlete gets up into the air in high jump also apply to other jumping skills (e.g., a volleyball spike, a basketball layup, and a receiver's leaping catch in football). Once in flight, the same mechanical laws apply to the long jumper (or any athlete in flight), as they do to the high jumper.
Throwing Striking Kicking	Javelin throw Baseball batting Football punting	All three skills require the athlete to generate high velocity. The javelin thrower wants the throwing hand moving as fast as possible, the baseball hitter wants the bat moving quickly, and the punter wants his foot moving at high velocity when it contacts the ball. In all three skills, athletes try to simulate a whiplash action with their limbs.
Pushing, pulling, lifting, and carrying	Clean and jerk	The clean is a lifting-pulling action and the jerk is a push. Carrying actions occur when the athlete pauses with the bar at the chest, and again when the bar is at arm's length above the head. The mechanical principles involved in the clean and jerk apply to all lifting, carrying, and spotting techniques. Laws controlling stability also play an important role in the clean and jerk.

General skill	Specific skill	Rationale
Swinging Rotating	Giant circle Front somersault	Swinging is a rotational skill controlled by many of the same mechanical principles that govern the front somersault. However, there are some differences. The giant circle is performed around a high bar, which acts as an axis external to the athlete's body. In contrast, the axis for a front somersault passes through the athlete's body from one hip to the other. There are similarities and differences in the mechanics of these two skills.
Equilibrium and stability	Judo hip throw	A judo hip throw represents the battle that occurs when athletes try to maintain their own stability and at the same time destroy the stability of their opponents. Judoka use pulling, pushing, and rotary actions to get their opponents off balance. The mechanical principles governing the giant circle, the front somersault, and the clean and jerk appear again in the judo hip throw.
Arresting motion	Judo breakfall	A judo breakfall demonstrates an athlete arresting the motion of his body. The principles that judoka apply in dissipating the forces that occur when they slam into the mat also apply when athletes catch balls, take hits in contact sports, and land after jumping. The breakfall is a technique used to increase the area and lengthen the time frame that impact forces are applied to the athletes' bodies when they drop on the mat.

Before You Start

As you read the following pages, look for mechanical principles that constantly reappear from one skill to the next! Watch for the turning effect of torque, the battle against inertia as athletes accelerate, and the athlete's use of impulse. It doesn't matter what skill you consider—these mechanical principles (and many others) are always present. Get to know them, to recognize them, and to understand their effect. It will help you immensely in your coaching.

Running Skills

Skill highlights

1. The time an athlete takes running over a set distance depends upon the athlete's stride length and stride frequency. The length of the athlete's legs and the forward thrust that occurs with each stride determine stride length. Forward thrust is produced by the earth's reaction force responding to the athlete's backward thrust against the earth's surface. Stride frequency is the cadence that the athlete uses (i.e., the number of strides that occurs each second).

2. A runner's technique changes the faster the athlete runs. Sprinters spend more time in the air than distance runners. In addition, they flex and swing their arms more vigorously. Sprinters also have a higher knee lift, a greater leg thrust, and a higher flexed leg. Distance runners use less arm action but tend to swing their shoulders more than sprinters. The longer the distance, the greater the reliance on cardiovascular endurance and pacing. All elite runners hold their torsos close to perpendicular.

3. Tension is detrimental to all runners because tension saps energy and restricts muscle action and limb movement. Sprinters try to run explosively while still relaxing their faces, necks, shoulders, and hands. Distance runners use the same relaxation techniques.

SPOTLIGHT ON . . .

Sprinting

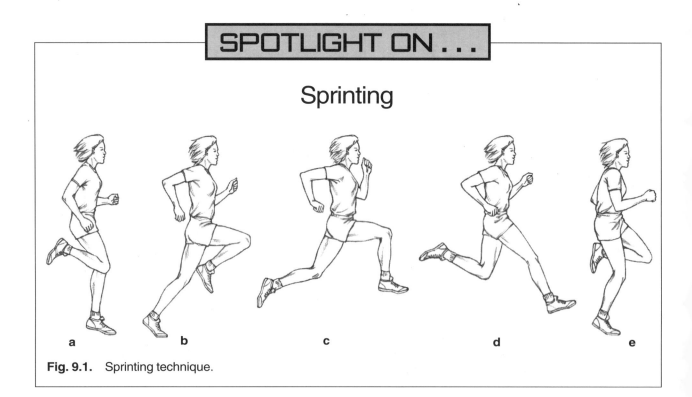

Fig. 9.1. Sprinting technique.

Sprinting

Technique	Mechanics
1. Good sprinting technique demands an optimal blend of stride length and stride frequency. A predominance of fast-twitch muscle fibers is essential for top-level sprinting.	1. A combination of optimal leg power, stride length, and stride frequency produces the best sprinting times. Power, good reactions, and excellent flexibility are all essential. Stride length depends on hip flexibility, leg length, muscle power, and range of movement. Training optimizes the forward thrust that occurs at each stride. Training also brings more muscle fibers into action and teaches the athlete to relax opposing muscle groups. Leg drive is improved by related power training. Overemphasis on stride frequency or on stride length produces inefficient sprinting.
2. Sprinting requires excellent leg, hip, and shoulder flexibility. Flexibility in the hip and pelvic area is particularly important.	2. An ability to rotate the hips around the long axis of the body helps to produce an optimal stride frequency and stride length. Flexibility in the shoulder girdle promotes good arm swing.
3. A sprinter's arms are flexed at 90 degrees and swing powerfully forward and backward. The hands are relaxed and swing hip high to the rear and shoulder high in front (see Figure 9.1, a-e).	3. Forward and backward arm swing counterbalances the twisting motion produced by each leg thrust on either side of the sprinter's long axis. Flexing the arms at the elbows reduces their rotary inertia and makes their pendular movement easier for the muscles involved. A vigorous forward swing of each arm transfers momentum to the athlete's body as a whole. This adds to the athlete's leg thrust and helps drive the athlete forward. Forward and backward arm swing (rather than across the body) helps to hold the torso and the shoulder girdle steady. This aids balance and relaxation, and assures that the athlete runs a straight line toward the finish.
4. The driving leg extends to near full extension (see Figure 9.1b). When the driving foot leaves the ground, the leg flexes and the heel kicks up to buttock level (see Figure 9.1e).	4. A powerful leg extension via the hip, knee, and ankle joints provides the athlete with optimal thrust in the direction of the sprint. Thrust backward and downward at 50 to 55 degrees produces an equal and opposite reaction from the earth, which drives the athlete in a predominately horizontal direction along the track. Flexion of the legs (like the arms) reduces their rotary inertia and makes their recovery and forward movement easier for the muscles involved.
5. After thrusting backward and downward, the driving leg flexes at the knee and is brought directly forward and upward so that the thigh swings to just below horizontal (see Figure 9.1c).	5. The swing and upward thrust of the driving leg as it is brought forward is counterbalanced by the action of the opposing arm. Forward thrust of both arm and leg generates momentum transfer. This helps produce a greater thrust back at the earth with the driving leg, and in response, from the earth propelling the sprinter's body along the track.

Sprinting

Technique	Mechanics
6. When the sprinter's driving leg is recovered and becomes the supporting leg, it flexes slightly on landing. The supporting foot lands below the sprinter's center of gravity. The first contact of the foot with the ground is on the outside edge of the foot. The heel is lowered but does not contact the track (see Figure 9.1e).	6. A slight flexion of the supporting leg extends the time of impact that force is applied to the sprinter's body and so cushions the landing. Flexion stretches the leg muscles, ready for extending the driving leg backward and downward against the earth. When the supporting foot lands below the sprinter's center of gravity, it eliminates deceleration that would occur if the foot was placed ahead of the sprinter's center of gravity.
7. A sprinter's forward body lean is extreme during a sprint start. At top speed the torso is perpendicular and the shoulder girdle held square to the direction of run (see Figure 9.1, a-e).	7. During a sprint start, forward body lean and shorter, high-frequency strides overcome the inertia of the sprinter's body mass and help the sprinter to gain momentum. At full speed, a perpendicular torso coupled with vigorous forward and backward arm action counterbalances the movement of the legs.
8. A sprinter's body rises and falls very little when running at full speed (see Figure 9.1, a-e).	8. An elite sprinter's center of gravity follows a low wavelike pattern as it travels forward. Slightly more time is spent in the air than in a support position. Too much time in the air is time wasted and indicates that too much thrust is directed vertically.
9. The sprinter's head is held in a natural alignment with the torso. Vision is horizontal and directly ahead (see Figure 9.1, a-e).	9. Proper position of the head and vision assists in maintaining the stability of the sprinter's torso. Tilting the head back increases tension and restricts stride frequency and stride length.
10. Good sprinting combines power with relaxation. Face, neck, shoulders, and hands are relaxed.	10. Tension in the body reduces the velocity of muscle contraction and reduces sprinting velocity. Good sprinting requires a rapid change from muscle contraction to relaxation. A technically superior sprinter is mechanically efficient. Unnecessary tension is avoided and in this way the athlete uses energy efficiently.
11. An athlete's sprinting speed is influenced by environmental conditions.	11. The greatest expenditure of energy in sprinting occurs when the athlete is thrusting back at the earth. Energy is also required for the knee lift and support phase of sprinting. The faster the athlete runs, the more energy the athlete must spend fighting air resistance. Headwinds add to this resistance. The condition of the track influences sprinting speed. Lightweight quality spikes producing good traction and driving back on a firm, rubberized track help to thrust the athlete forward better than running on soft ground.

Swimming Skills

Skill highlights

1. The velocity with which a swimmer moves through the water depends on stroke length and stroke frequency. The reaction forces of the water responding to the forces that the swimmer applies against the water produce stroke length (i.e., the distance traveled with each stroke). Stroke frequency refers to the number of strokes per minute.

2. A swimmer's hands and arms produce the greatest propulsive forces in swimming. These propulsive forces occur predominately because of lift and drag forces generated by propellerlike sculling and blading actions. Propulsive forces are greatest when sculling and blading occurs in nonturbulent, still water containing a minimum of air bubbles.

3. Swimmers must fight form drag, surface drag, and wave drag. A horizontal body position combined with smooth surfaces (caused by shaving and the use of slick swimsuit fabrics) reduce form and surface drag to minimal levels. Swimmers counteract wave drag (and air bubbles) by reducing up and down body motion and by eliminating slapping arm entries.

SPOTLIGHT ON . . .

Front Crawl

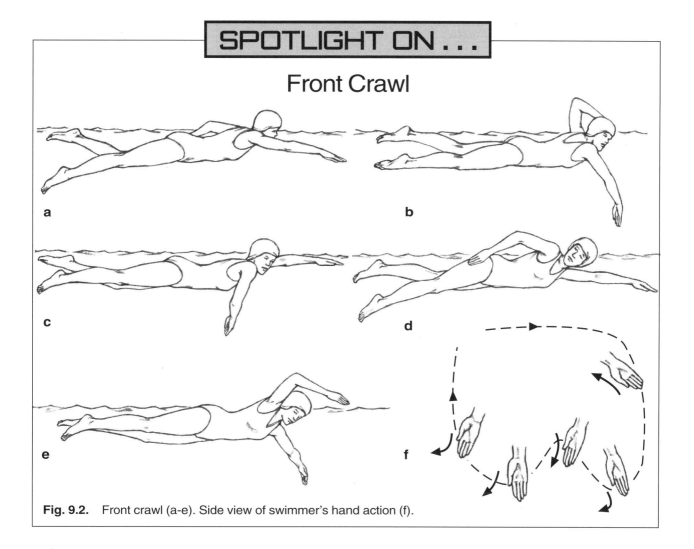

Fig. 9.2. Front crawl (a-e). Side view of swimmer's hand action (f).

Front Crawl

Technique	Mechanics
1. The front crawl is the fastest of the four swimming strokes. The front crawl synchronizes arm action, leg kick, general body position, and breathing.	1. In the front crawl, one arm pulls while the other recovers. The front and back crawl use this cyclic action, whereas the breaststroke and butterfly pull and recover both arms at the same time. Breathing, leg kick, and arm action are synchronized and rhythmic. The arms, and particularly the hands, produce most of the propulsive force in the front crawl.
2. The swimmer's face is in the water with the water level at the hairline and the body lying horizontally. The head turns but is not raised for breathing. The feet kick just below the surface. The recovery of the arms as they are brought forward follows a line parallel to the long axis of the swimmer's body (see Figure 9.2, a-e).	2. Raising the head causes the legs to drop and generate drag. Kicking too deep also increases drag. Swinging the arms across the body as they reach forward to enter the water destroys alignment and causes the body to move in the opposing direction. This generates excessive form drag. Some body roll along the long axis during the forward reach of the arms helps maintain lateral alignment and reduce drag.
3. During its recovery, the arm is flexed at the elbow. Entry is made ahead of the head at a position between the midline of the head and the shoulder joint. At entry, the arm flexes slightly with the elbow above the hand. Fingertips slice into the water before any other part of the hand and arm.	3. A flexed arm during the recovery reduces its rotary inertia making it easier for the muscles involved to bring the arm forward. Slamming the hand into the water causes the body to react in the opposing motion and to bounce up and down. A slapping entry causes waves and air bubbles. Both increase drag, which resists the movement of the swimmer.
4. The propulsive phase of each stroke starts from an outstretched arm as the hand is slid forward under the water. The fingertips extend the line of the forearm. The forward reach of the arm occurs at the same time the opposing arm finishes the upward sweep of its pulling action (see Figure 9.2d).	4. A long, extended reach and pull by the swimmer increases the impulse (i.e., the distance over which the force of the pull occurs). The synchronized cyclic action of the arms maintains the swimmer's momentum. It requires more muscular force (and energy) if the swimmer repetitively accelerates and decelerates with each arm pull.
5. A blading-sculling motion with the pulling hand is the predominant propulsive action. From entry through to exit, the hand follows an S-shaped outsweep, downsweep, insweep, and upsweep motion. The hand is angled and pitched throughout to simulate the blading motion of a propeller. Some propulsion is gained by pushing directly back against the water (see Figure 9.2f).	5. Propulsion in the crawl results from lift and drag forces that come from sculling and blading with the hands. The correct angle of attack (varying between 20 and 40 degrees relative to the water flowing past the hand) is necessary. Some propulsive force occurs because of pushing back on the water, and the water in reaction pushing the swimmer forward. Too much emphasis on pushing against the water like a paddlewheeler is incorrect.

Front Crawl

Technique	Mechanics
6. During their blading and sculling action, the swimmer's hands search for still, nonturbulent water, which contains minimal air bubbles.	6. The greatest propulsive force in the crawl stroke is generated by the hands. Additional help is gained from the active surfaces of the arms. Lift forces are greatest when sculling and blading occurs in nonturbulent, still water, which contains little to no air bubbles.
7. Just beyond the midpoint in the pull, the arm flexes at the elbow. The elbow is high, and in relation the hand is positioned lower in the water (see Figure 9.2 c). The degree of flexion at the elbow differs from one phase to another within the crawl stroke.	7. Flexion reduces the resistance arm of the pulling arm making it easier for the swimmer's muscles to pull it along its elliptical pathway. The active surface area of the hand and arm is not reduced when the arm is flexed.
8. The crawl swimmer's hand accelerates as it moves through its outsweep, downsweep, insweep, and upsweep motion. Maximum velocity is reached at the end of the upsweep.	8. A smooth, continuous acceleration of the hand during its pull increases the propulsive forces generated. This action increases the velocity of the swimmer through the water.
9. The flutter kick is 1 to 2 ft deep and occurs just below the surface of the water (see Figure 9.2, a-e). It has a downbeat, upbeat, plus some lateral motion. The downbeat is initiated before the same leg has totally finished its upbeat. The kick starts at the hip and works down to the ankle in a whiplash motion. The flutter kick is synchronized with the arm action.	9. The flutter kick adds little to propulsion but holds the swimmer's body in a streamlined horizontal position. Up and down flutter action provide an equal contribution. Kicking too deep increases drag without contributing to propulsion. Some lateral motion in the kick helps to stabilize the body as it rolls for each arm stroke. Flexibility at the ankle is particularly important. The width of the kick depends on the swimmer's build, strength, and stroke rate. A stiff-legged flutter kick is energy consuming and incorrect.
10. The number of flutter kicks per stroke cycle can be 2, 4, or 6. The upward and downward kick is synchronized with the out-sweep, downsweep, insweep, and upsweep arm action.	10. The frequency of stroke and leg kick is greatest in the short sprints and lowest in distance swimming. Vigorous 6-beat kicking is energy consuming, but often used by less buoyant males to help maintain an efficient horizontal body position during short distance races. The 4-beat kick is used as an energy-saving kick while still maintaining good lateral and horizontal body alignment. A 2-beat kick is often used over long distances because it demands less energy. Females are generally more buoyant than males and often use a 2-beat kick. Swimmers temporarily increase the number of leg beats when accelerating away from the wall of the pool after completing a tumble-turn.
11. Excellent flexibility and joint mobility help to maximize propulsion and to maintain an efficient body position in the water.	11. Flexibility and joint mobility, particularly in the shoulders, hips, knees, and ankles, increase the range over which forces are generated and help to reduce nonproductive drag forces.

Jumping Skills

Skill highlights

1. To get up in the air, jumpers exert a force against the earth's surface well in excess of their own body weight. The earth's reaction force then drives the athletes upward. The more forceful the athlete's thrust against the earth, the greater the earth's response.

2. Immediately before takeoff, a jumper's center of gravity is lowered, the body tilted backward, and the athlete's arms and free leg positioned to the rear of the body. Lowering the body prestretches the big muscles of the jumping leg ready for the leg's explosive thrust downward at the earth. Leaning back combines with lowering the body so the athlete can spend more time over the jumping foot applying force to the earth. Swinging the arms forward and upward adds to the downward thrust of the athlete's jumping leg against the earth.

3. The path that a jumper's center of gravity follows during flight is determined by the velocity that the athlete is propelled upward at takeoff, and (a) the takeoff angle used.

4. When in flight, movement of one part of a jumper's body causes other parts to move in the opposing direction. In high jump, this characteristic helps in bar clearance. In long jump, rotary actions of the arms and legs are used in flight to counteract the unwanted forward rotation that inevitably occurs when the athlete takes off. In a volleyball spike, drawing the arm back and arching the body in a counterclockwise direction will cause the legs to move in a clockwise direction.

SPOTLIGHT ON . . .

Flop High Jump

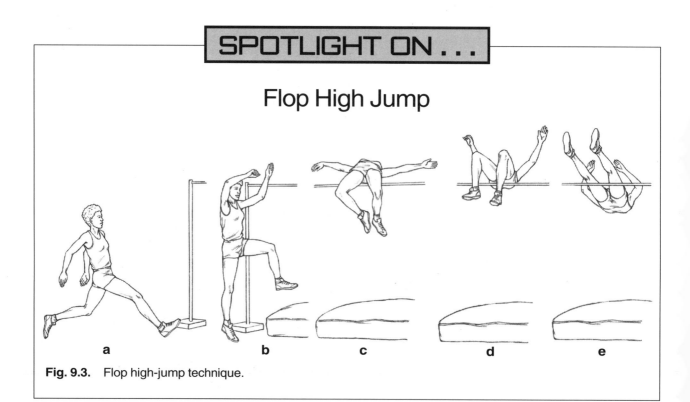

a   b   c   d   e

Fig. 9.3. Flop high-jump technique.

Flop High Jump

Technique	Mechanics
1. Run-ups used by elite athletes in the flop high jump range from 10 to 13 strides and commonly extend over a curved approach of 60 to 80 ft. Flop jumpers approach the bar at high velocity and accelerate to even greater velocity during the last 3 strides before takeoff.	1. A flop high jump run-up should be long enough so that a velocity is reached that is sufficient to carry the athlete through the actions performed at takeoff.
2. The greater the velocity of the run-up, the greater its potential in helping the athlete to jump high. Too much or too little velocity in the run-up can be detrimental to the takeoff.	2. The greater the velocity of the run-up, the greater its tendency to shorten the time during which force is exerted by the athlete against the ground at takeoff. The faster the run-up the greater the need for superb leg power and coordination during the takeoff. There is no benefit in a faster run-up if an athlete lacks the physical ability to use its additional velocity.
3. Most flop high jumpers use a curved run-up that has a large radius curve (or is almost straight) during the first six to seven strides, followed by a small radius curve during the final three to five strides. Flop jumpers lean into the curve of the run-up. They also lean backward as they plant the takeoff foot (see Figure 9.3a).	3. The athlete's inward lean during the run-up produces a centripetal force. A tighter curve requires more inward lean. Inward and backward lean as the jumping foot is planted lengthens the time that the athlete spends thrusting down at the earth with the jumping leg. Inward and backward lean before takeoff counterbalance the outward pull of inertia and centrifugal force. A body position with lean away from the bar prevents the athlete from committing the error of leaning into (i.e., toward) the bar.
4. During the last two to three strides of the run-up the athlete's center of gravity is lowered and the arms and free leg positioned to the rear of the body (see Figure 9.3a). The penultimate (i.e., next to last) stride and the final stride are longer than those that occur prior. The athlete steps forward onto the jumping foot with the hips positioned well to the rear of the jumping foot.	4. Lowering the center of gravity and stepping well forward onto the jumping foot allows the athlete to apply force against the earth over a large arc (i.e., a long time frame) and in reaction have the earth spend more time driving the athlete upward. Lowering the center of gravity prestretches the jumping muscles in preparation for their powerful extension of the jumping leg.
5. The arms and free leg are positioned to the rear of the body as the athlete steps forward onto the jumping leg (see Figure 9.3a). The forward and upward swing of the arms and free leg is coordinated with the extension of the jumping leg (see Figure 9.3b).	5. The upward swing of the arms and the free leg toward the bar is a form of momentum transfer. The momentum of their upward swing combines with the downward thrust of the takeoff leg. All unify to produce a greater reactive response from the earth, which drives the athlete upward.

Flop High Jump

Technique	Mechanics
6. The free leg and arms flex and accelerate during their upward swing. These actions occur while the takeoff leg is extending vigorously in contact with the earth (see Figure 9.3b).	6. Flexing the arms and legs brings their mass closer to their respective axes and reduces their rotary inertia. This action makes it easier for the athlete's muscles to move them upward at high speed. For greatest effect the free leg and arms move at maximum velocity at that instant when the athlete is last in contact with the earth. The muscles in the jumping leg must have enough power to extend the jumping leg explosively.
7. The takeoff for elite flop jumpers is from a point 3 to 4 ft directly out from the near high jump standard. The takeoff foot is placed at an angle of 15 to 20 degrees to the cross bar. The free leg is first thrust upward and then rotated away from the bar and back toward the run-up. The shoulders rotate parallel to the bar. Vision is usually along the bar in the direction of the far standard.	7. Rotation of the jumper's body into a back-lying position over the bar is initiated while the takeoff foot is still in contact with the ground. The athlete is then able to rotate around the body's long axis by pushing against the earth's surface. In the air, the same movement causes a twistlike equal and opposite reaction to occur. Elite jumpers try not to compromise vertical thrust by overemphasizing rotation during the takeoff.
8. At takeoff the high velocity of the run-up coupled with the plant of the takeoff foot causes the athlete to move forward over the takeoff foot.	8. Moving up and over the takeoff foot initiates rotation, which continues in flight. Once in flight the athlete can rotate more quickly (i.e., increase his or her angular velocity) by pulling the body inward, or slow down rotation by stretching out and extending the body.
9. After takeoff the athlete's upper body is flexed backward over the bar. The free (i.e., leading) leg, which was swung up at the bar, is lowered from its elevated position (see Figure 9.3c).	9. Lowering the leading leg, combined with the act of flexing the upper body backward, produces an equal and opposite reaction that elevates the athlete's hips. This clears the hips over the bar. The athlete's vision, directed along the length of the bar, helps to time this critical maneuver.
10. When the athlete's seat has crossed the bar, the head and shoulders are lifted upward. The athlete's torso and the legs (which are now flexed at the knee) are pulled toward each other by the contraction of the abdominal and quadriceps muscles (see Figure 9.3d).	10. The elevation of the head and shoulders causes two equal and opposite reactions to occur: (1) The flexed legs move upward toward the torso, and (2) the athlete's seat (which has crossed the bar) drops downward. Flexion of the legs reduces their rotary inertia making their movement easier so they are quickly drawn over the bar.

Flop High Jump

Technique	Mechanics
11. Once the athlete's thighs have cleared the bar, the legs are extended so that the heels avoid clipping the bar (see Figure 9.3e).	11. Even though the legs extend, the fact that the athlete's upper and lower body have moved toward each other causes the athlete's body to increase its rate of spin (angular velocity) around the athlete's transverse (hip to hip) axis. This action, combined with some rotation around the long axis continues as the jumper drops toward the pit.
12. The athlete relaxes to drop onto the shoulders on the high jump landing pad.	12. The continued rotation of the athlete's body in flight causes the athlete to drop onto the shoulders on the landing pad. The focus of the eyes on the bar during the clearance of the feet pulls the chin into the chest and prevents a head-first landing. The height of the high jump landing pad relative to the bar is designed to stop overrotation and prevent the athlete landing on the back of the neck. The foam rubber of the landing pads extends the time frame and area of impact and gradually reduces the forces applied to the athlete during the landing.

Throwing, Striking, and Kicking Skills

Skill highlights

1. In high-velocity throwing and striking skills, there is a rapid acceleration of the athlete's body segments, beginning with those in contact with the earth. This whiplike, or flail-like sequence progresses upward from the legs to the hips, from hips to chest, and culminates in the tremendous velocity of the striking or throwing arm. To achieve the greatest possible velocity, it is important that antagonist muscle groups are completely relaxed.

2. Kicking skills differ from throwing and striking skills in that the last and fastest moving links in the whiplike sequence are the athlete's lower leg and kicking foot. The progressive acceleration of body segments in kicking skills is similar to that of throwing and striking skills.

3. Each movement pattern in throwing, striking, and kicking skills contains a preparatory action commonly called a windup or backswing. A windup provides additional distance over which force is applied. It also prestretches the athlete's muscles ready for their explosive recoil. Relaxation and flexibility help to produce an optimal windup.

SPOTLIGHT ON . . .

Javelin Throw

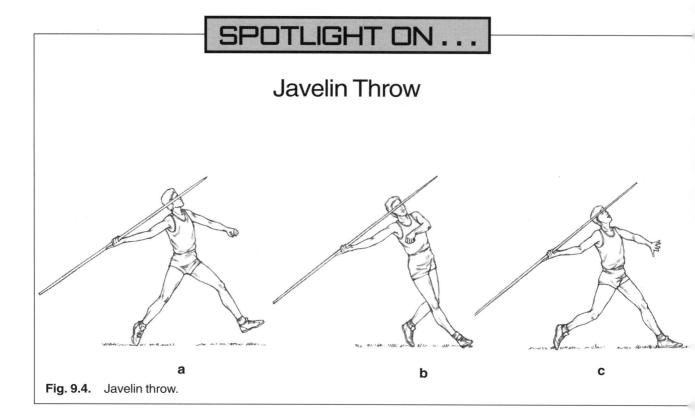

a   b   c

Fig. 9.4.   Javelin throw.

Javelin Throw

Technique	Mechanics
1. A run-up toward the direction of throw leads into a wide powerful throwing stance. The run-up is relaxed and increases in velocity. The athlete accelerates during the first two thirds of the approach. This leads into the final one third of the throw, which includes the withdrawal of the javelin and the final throwing motion.	1. A run-up builds momentum and generates enough velocity to carry the athlete through the throwing stance and into the follow-through. Too much velocity in the early part of the run-up may cause the athlete either to slow down during the throwing actions, or conversely not allow enough time in the throwing stance to apply an optimal amount of force to the javelin. Efficient use of a run-up can increase the distance thrown by 90 to 100 ft compared with a standing throw.
2. Before entering the throwing stance, the athlete's shoulder girdle is rotated away from the direction of throw, and the throwing arm is taken back to arm's length (see Figure 9.4a). By use of one or more crossover steps, the lower body moves forward under the torso so the athlete's body is angled backward away from the direction of throw (see Figure 9.4, a-b).	2. The purpose of the rotation of the shoulder girdle coupled with the extension of the throwing arm is to prepare the athlete for the application of force over the largest possible distance and time frame. The backward body lean makes this distance and time frame even greater.

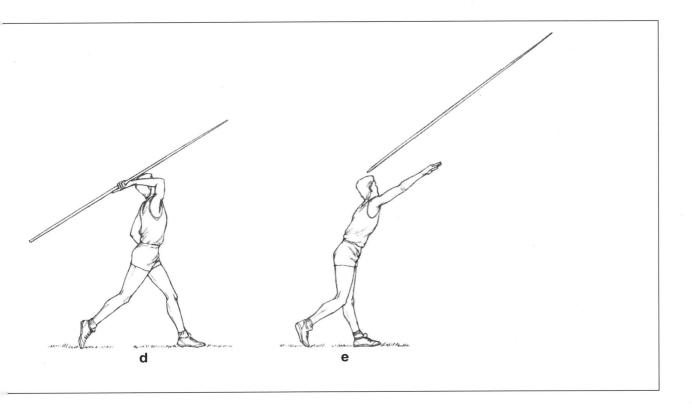

d   e

Javelin Throw

Technique	Mechanics
3. The athlete steps into the throwing stance with the leg on the opposite side of the body to the throwing arm. This step is considerably larger than those prior (see Figure 9.4c).	3. Stepping forward with the opposing foot sets up a large base of support for the application of force. This allows the athlete's hips and shoulders to be rotated away from the direction of throw.
4. The athlete's body is tilted backward and the center of gravity lowered over a partially flexed rear leg. The rear leg is flexed at the knee and angled 45 degrees from the direction of throw.	4. Flexing the rear leg stretches the leg muscles in preparation for their explosive rotary thrust toward the direction of throw. This rotary motion is the first stage in the athlete's whiplash action that starts from the athlete's base and progresses up to the throwing arm.
5. The rear leg is vigorously rotated toward the direction of throw. This action thrusts the hips in the same direction (See Figure 9.4, c-d). The muscles joining the hips to the torso stretch and contract explosively.	5. More massive, slower moving parts of the body shift forward into the throw while lighter body segments (e.g., the throwing arm) complete their backward extension. This motion stretches the muscles in the abdomen, chest, and shoulders ready for their explosive contraction during later phases of the throw.
6. The athlete's torso rotates and pulls the shoulders and the throwing arm toward the direction of throw. Opposing muscle groups	6. Each of the athlete's body segments, from the legs through to the shoulders and throwing arm, sequentially accelerate. This sequence sets up a flail-like

Javelin Throw

Technique	Mechanics
are relaxed. As the shoulders are pulled forward, the muscles of the shoulders stretch and then contract vigorously. A relaxed throwing arm follows the shoulder with a flail-like action. The athlete's body tilts sideways away from the throwing arm. The free arm rotates backward to help pull the chest and throwing arm around and into the throw (see Figure 9.4, c-d).	whip-cracking action that progressively builds and ends in the tremendous velocity of the throwing arm. A sideways inclination of the athlete's body allows for greater height of release. The free arm is pulled backward to help rotate the athlete's torso around the long axis of the body. Rotation of the torso makes a contribution in pulling the throwing arm at high velocity into the throw.
7. As the athlete's throwing arm is pulled forward, the upper arm and elbow lead with the throwing hand and javelin trailing well behind. Flexion occurs at the elbow of the throwing arm (see Figure 9.4d).	7. Flexing the throwing arm at the elbow serves two purposes: (1) It helps the athlete to become even more whiplike, and (2) the elbow acts like the axle of a wheel with the throwing hand rotating around at its rim. This wheel-axle arrangement increases the velocity of the throwing hand and the javelin.
8. The athlete thrusts forward toward the direction of throw. The torso moves forward beyond the supporting leg, which has been straightened (see Figure 9.4e).	8. Forcefully driving the body as far as possible toward the direction of throw extends the application of force to the javelin over the longest possible distance and time period.
9. The athlete uses a follow-through to complete the throw (see Figure 9.4e).	9. The follow-through applies force to the javelin for as long as possible. After the javelin has left the athlete's hand, the follow-through allows for safe dissipation of momentum from the athlete's body.
10. The angle of release of the javelin varies according to the throwing ability of the athlete, the type of javelin used, and environmental conditions at the time of throwing.	10. A javelin is dramatically affected by lift and drag forces. The trajectory angle and the position of the javelin at release relative to environmental conditions, such as head- and tailwinds, all determine the flight path and the distance that the javelin follows.

SPOTLIGHT ON...

Baseball Batting

Technique	Mechanics
1. In baseball, a batter faces an approaching ball that is usually spinning and varies in velocity and direction. A baseball bat is cylindrical and has a curved striking surface. Hitting the ball effectively is extremely difficult. Fastballs can have velocities of close to, and even over, 100 mph. Batters have less than a second to react to the pitch.	1. When a batter wants to strike a ball and send it in the opposing direction, the momentum of the bat must be greater than that of the ball. Arm extension, club length, and the rate of swing determine the velocity of the barrel end of the bat. Timing and coordination are essential for hitting the ball through its center of gravity, rather than hitting it off center (i.e., out of line with the ball's center of gravity) and producing a pop-up.
2. Batters take a stance that is slightly larger than shoulder width. Their body weight is close to, or over the rear foot, which is at right angles to the approaching pitch. Right-handed batters stand with the left side and left hip toward the pitcher. The head is turned so that the batter can concentrate on the pitcher's actions. The bat is frequently held in a ready position with the barrel end pointing skyward (see Figure 9.5a)	2. The initial shoulder-width stance with the body weight above the rear foot allows the batter to shift the center of gravity forward an optimal distance into the hitting stance. With the left side facing the pitcher, right-handed batters can rotate their hips and torsos more than 90 degrees as part of the batting action. Moving the body toward the pitch (plus rotating the hips and torso) increases the distance over which force is applied to the bat and subsequently to the ball.
3. As the ball approaches the plate, right-handed batters step approximately an additional half-shoulder width toward the pitcher. This puts them into a wide, powerful, hitting stance. The batter's arms extend partially away from the body. There is commonly some backward rotation of the shoulders and the bat as the batter shifts forward toward the ball (see Figure 9.5b).	3. Movement of the batter's body mass toward the pitch stretches the muscles that subsequently pull the bat around toward the ball. The trailing action of the shoulders, arms, and bat in relation to the movement of the batter's hips will set up a whiplash action characteristic of high velocity throwing, kicking, and striking skills. Body rotation, coupled with arm extension, increases the angular velocity of the bat.
4. As the batter (right-handed) shifts forward from the right rear foot toward the left, the hips rotate around an axis formed by the left side of the body and the left leg. This action begins with turning in the rear knee and rotating on both feet toward the pitcher. The exact pathway followed by the bat is determined by the batter when reacting to the flight path of the pitch (see Figure 9.5, b-c).	4. The batter initiates the sequential rotation of the legs, hips, torso from the ground up. More massive body segments (i.e. legs, hips, torso), are vigorously rotated, then suddenly decelerated. Their angular velocity is multiplied up through the batter's body and along the length of the batter's arms out to the barrel section of the bat. The bat rotates in flail-like fashion around axes formed by the left shoulder and the batter's wrists.

Baseball Batting

Technique	Mechanics
5. When the bat is swung around at high velocity, the batter is forced to lean backward away from the bat.	5. The tremendous angular velocity of the bat requires that the batter generate considerable centripetal force. The batter leans away from the bat and in doing so combines lean with gravity's downward pull on his body mass to counterbalance the inertial and centrifugal pull of the bat.
6. The batter attempts to strikes the ball at the bat's sweet spot. To drive the ball a great distance, the batter tries to avoid a slicing impact, and instead, to hit the ball through its center.	6. It is best if the batter strike the ball at the bat's center of percussion (i.e., the bat's sweet spot). If the force applied by the bat fails to pass through the ball's center of gravity, the ball can be undercut and given backspin. A magnus effect is applied to the ball counteracting gravity and giving it lift. The ball hangs up in the air making it an easy target for a fielder. An overcut will give the ball topspin. In this case the magnus effect joins gravity's downward pull and the ball arcs quickly down toward the earth.

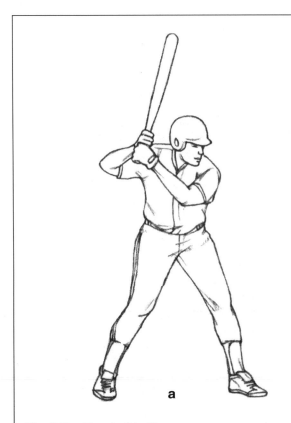
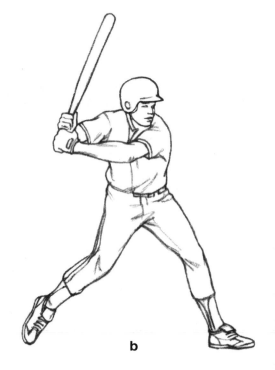

Fig. 9.5. Baseball batting.

Baseball Batting

Technique	Mechanics
7. The batter's arms swing forward and away from the chest. The left arm will extend as the bat swings around the body into the follow-through. The batter rotates around the left leg and the left side of the body (see Figure 9.5d). Vision is on the flight of the ball.	7. The batter's body rotates around the axis of the left side of the body. This extends the radius of rotation from the left shoulder out to the barrel of the bat. A follow-through completes the striking action and dissipates the momentum built up in the rotary action of the batter's body and the bat.
8. The flight of the ball depends on what occurs when the ball is hit plus the effect of environmental conditions.	8. The velocity, direction, and distance that the ball travels after it is hit depend on a large number of factors. These factors include the following: (a) The momentum of the ball at the instant of impact (b) The momentum of the bat at the instant of impact (c) The elasticity (recoil) of the ball (d) The direction that the bat and ball are moving at the instant of impact (e) The point of impact between the bat and the ball (f) The spin put on the ball after impact (g) Environmental conditions such as altitude, temperature, humidity, and airflow.

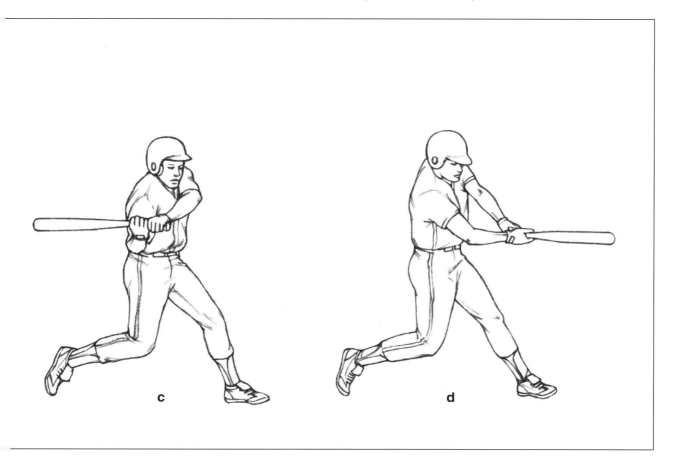

c   d

SPOTLIGHT ON . . .

Football Punting

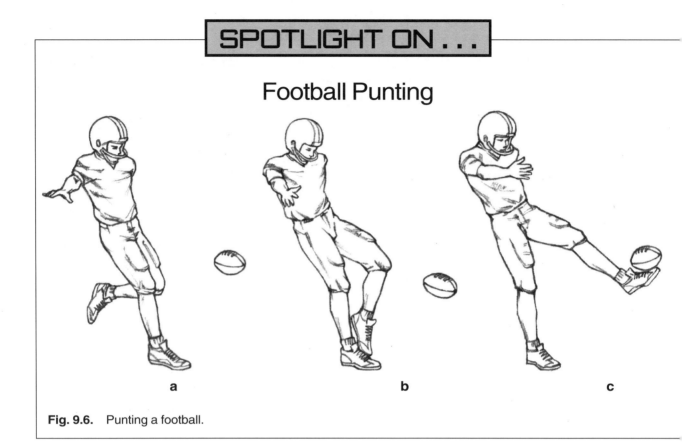

a   b   c

Fig. 9.6. Punting a football.

Football Punting

Technique	Mechanics
1. Kicking is a striking action used to apply force with the foot. Punting a football uses the kicking leg in much the same way a javelin thrower uses the throwing arm, or a batter uses both arms and a bat to strike a baseball.	1. Punting relates mechanically to striking actions made with a club or bat. It also relates mechanically to throwing actions in which the object thrown is lightweight and moves at high velocity. Kicking also requires the athlete to simulate the actions of a whip. Long legs, great muscular strength, and a huge range of movement help to generate a tremendous impact force when the kicking foot contacts the ball.
2. An athlete punts a football by stepping forward onto the supporting foot. This foot is positioned in front of the athlete's body, which is inclined backward (see Figure 9.6a). The kicker's arms extend forward so the ball is held well ahead of the body and fed onto the kicking foot. Vision is on the ball.	2. In punting, an athlete overcomes the inertia of his body (and that of the ball) by moving forward toward the direction of kick. This gives momentum both to the athlete and the ball. The supporting foot is placed well ahead of the athlete's center of gravity so that the athlete can move forward, up, over, and beyond this foot, which acts as an axis. The athlete's forward movement extends the time frame that force is applied to the ball.

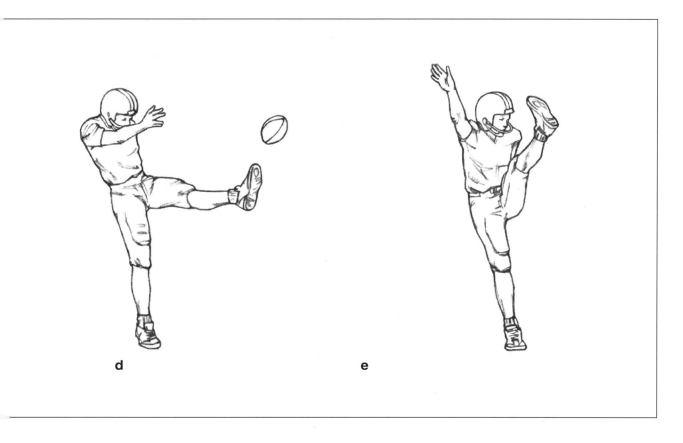

d   e

Football Punting

Technique	Mechanics
3. As the athlete steps into the kicking stance, the kicking leg (which is flexed at the knee) trails well to the rear of the athlete's body (see Figure 9.6a).	3. The trailing action of the kicking leg and the backward tilt of the athlete's body extends the time and distance that force is applied to the ball. The kicking foot travels over a huge arc from its backswing position to the point where it contacts the ball.
4. As the thigh of the kicking leg is swung forward, the lower leg trails to the rear and temporarily rotates in the opposing direction. A 90-degree angle occurs at the knee (see Figure 9.6b).	4. The forward swing of the thigh and the backward motion of the lower leg simulate the initial action of a whip, where the more massive lower part of the whip moves forward while lighter sections momentarily move in the opposing direction.
5. After accelerating forward and upward, the thigh of the kicking leg slows down. The lower leg and kicking foot now accelerate. The athlete will have positioned the ball ahead of the body so the kicking foot meets it while moving at high velocity.	5. The high angular velocity of the thigh is arrested. This causes its angular velocity to be passed onto the lower leg, which is less massive and has less rotary resistance. The angular velocity of the lower leg is dramatically increased. The ball is positioned so the impact occurs when the kicking foot has maximum momentum.

Football Punting

Technique	**Mechanics**
6. The kicking leg is extended when it contacts the ball (see Figure 9.6c).	6. There is a powerful extension of the kicking leg as the lower leg rotates around the axis of the knee joint. The kicking foot, simulating the tip of the whip, now moves at maximum velocity.
7. The athlete rises up on an extended supporting leg. The athlete's body tilts backward away from the direction of punt (see Figure 9.6, d-e).	7. Rising onto the toes of an extended supporting leg coupled with a backward body tilt enlarges the arc through which the kicking leg swings and force is applied to the ball.
8. The athlete's body moves forward past the supporting foot and in the direction of the kick. After the foot contacts the ball, the kicking leg continues with a follow-through. Flexion reoccurs at the knee of the kicking leg.	8. Forward movement of the athlete's body continues the application of force to the ball. Maximum angular velocity of the lower part of the kicking leg occurs just before contact with the ball. Partial flexion of the kicking leg allows the foot to swing upward through a large arc to a position above the athlete's head. The arms are often extended sideways to maintain stability.
9. The distance the ball travels depends on: (a) how much force is applied to the ball, (b) the trajectory angle of the ball, (c) environmental conditions, and (d) whether the ball spirals around its long axis or tumbles end over end.	9. The velocity of the kicking foot at the instant it contacts the ball, coupled with the angle of release, determines the distance the ball travels. Feeding the ball onto the kicking foot so it has a high trajectory angle when contact is made is used when kicking with a following wind. A low trajectory angle is used when kicking against the wind.
10. For a spiraling kick, the athlete positions the ball so its long axis is slightly offset from the intended direction of kick. The kicking foot is swung directly ahead and is drawn across the long axis of the ball.	10. Contacting the ball so the kicking foot moves across the long axis of the ball applies torque to the ball causing it to spin around its long axis. A spiraling ball will have greater stability and travel a greater distance than a ball that tumbles end over end.

Pulling, Pushing, Lifting, and Carrying Skills

Skill highlights

1. Sports that use push-pull actions (e.g., rowing, kayaking, archery, and weight lifting) require the athlete to apply force continuously throughout the desired range of movement. If an athlete wants to apply maximum force to a heavy resistance, the athlete simultaneously uses the largest number of body segments that can be applied to the task (i.e., the legs, back, chest, shoulders, and arms). This simultaneous action differs from high-velocity throwing, kicking, and striking skills in which a sequential movement of body segments occurs.

2. Spotting in gymnastics is a lifting-carrying motion. It requires the line of gravity of the performer to be as close as possible to that of the spotters. The faster the performer moves, the larger the performer's body mass, and the greater the distance from the spotter, the greater the oppositional or resistive torque produced by the performer! Spotters must counter this torque by moving as close to the performer as possible.

SPOTLIGHT ON . . .

Clean and Jerk

Technique	Mechanics
1. The two Olympic weight-lifting events are the clean and jerk and the snatch. The clean and jerk is used to hoist the heaviest poundages and is a two-phase lift. The bar is first pulled to the chest where a pause occurs. The athlete then jerks (pushes) the bar to arm's length above the head. The snatch differs from the clean and jerk in that it is performed with a continuous pulling action with no pause at the chest.	1. The clean and jerk and the snatch are both power events in which strength and speed are combined. In these events the athlete applies great force in a limited time frame to accelerate the barbell upward. At the height of the barbell's upward movement, the athlete must move at high speed into positions where the barbell is stabilized at the chest (for the clean) and above the head for the jerk and the snatch.
2. The clean and jerk uses two types of leg action. With a heavy barbell, an athlete cleans the bar by first pulling on it and lifting it as high as possible. Without pause, the athlete either squats under the bar or splits the legs forward and backward. The athlete then rises up out of this position with the bar positioned at the chest ready for the jerk. To complete the jerk, an upward jerking action occurs which is combined with a lunge motion in which the legs are split forward and backward.	2. The quicker the bar moves upward, and the higher it travels, the more time available for the athlete to perform the squat or leg split. The more powerful the athlete (and/or the lighter the resistance), the faster and higher will be the upward movement of the bar. A bar pulled upward to a high position does not require a high-speed performance of a deep squat or a leg split as the athlete moves under the bar.

Clean and Jerk

Technique	Mechanics
3. The starting position in the clean has the athlete in a shoulder-width stance with the bar in front of the shins. The athlete grips the bar with the hands slightly wider than shoulder-width and equidistant from the plates. The arms and back are straight and the legs flexed no more than necessary. The athlete's back is angled at 45 degrees to the horizontal (see Figure 9.7a).	3. The starting position for the clean is such that the bar will be pulled predominately in a vertical manner. The athlete's partially flexed legs (e.g., approximately a half squat) are in a mechanically efficient position for a powerful extension. The arms are extended and immediately transmit force from the athlete's legs and back to the bar.
4. The clean begins with the bar being accelerated upward by a powerful extension of the athlete's legs and back.	4. The resting inertia of the bar is overcome by a powerful extension of the athlete's legs and back. Both legs and back extend simultaneously, transferring the pull to the bar via the arms. The bar rises in a vertical direction.
5. When the legs have completed their extension, the athlete continues to pull upward by flexing the arms. The athlete rises up onto the toes and hyperextends the back. The pull of the arms completes the vertical movement of the bar, which travels upward close to the athlete's body. The head is thrown back (see Figure 9.7b).	5. The large muscles of the legs and back apply the greatest force to the bar. Driving up onto the toes and pulling upward with the arms allows the athlete to continue applying force to the bar over a long time frame. The athlete pulls the bar upward as close to his line of gravity as possible. In this way the center of gravity of the bar stays above (and within) the athlete's supporting base and the athlete and bar are optimally stabilized.

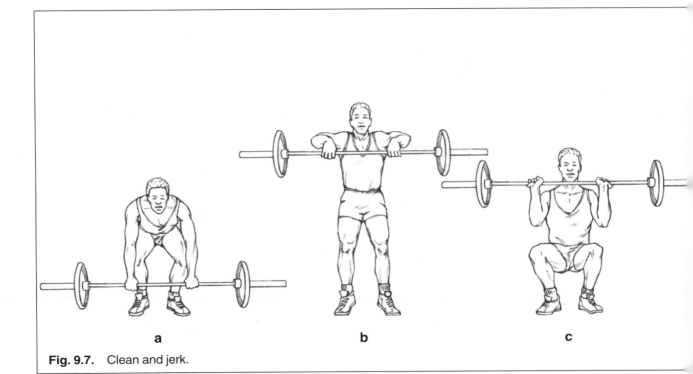

a   b   c

Fig. 9.7. Clean and jerk.

Clean and Jerk

Technique	Mechanics
6. When the barbell has risen to just below the pectoral muscles, the athlete squats down under the bar, simultaneously rotating the arms forward so the bar is pulled in toward the upper chest and held in place by the arms (see Figure 9.7c).	6. The greater the mass (weight) of the barbell, the more critical becomes the upward pull on the bar, and likewise the velocity with which the athlete rotates the arms forward and squats under the bar. A sufficiently high pull, coupled with fast arm rotation and equally fast squatting action, are absolutely essential.
7. The athlete uses the great strength in the legs to lift up from a deep front squat position (see Figure 9.7c-d).	7. With the bar at the chest and in a deep squat, the athlete must use the great strength in his legs to battle the deadweight (i.e., inertia) of the barbell (plus the inertia of his own body mass) so he can rise to a standing position. With insufficient strength and/or too massive (i.e., too heavy) a barbell, the athlete will either (a) fail to get up out of the squat, or (b) be physically drained from the effort of standing up, and fail to complete the jerk.
8. In a standing position and with the bar held at the chest, the athlete dips and flexes the legs slightly. The weight discs at either end of the bar cause the bar to flex downward then upward.	8. A slight flexion prestretches the leg muscles before the extension of the legs. The upward recoil of the bar is timed to coincide with the leg extension to assist in thrusting the barbell upward.

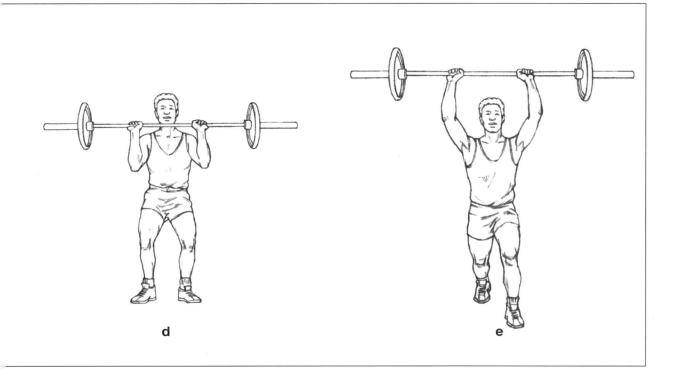

d   e

Clean and Jerk

Technique	Mechanics
9. The instant the athlete's legs have completed their thrust and the bar is rising upward, the legs split forward and backward. One leg is extended directly backward at an angle of about 45 degrees. The opposite foot steps forward 8 to 10 in. This allows the athlete to lunge forward under the bar (see Figure 9.7e).	9. The athlete's leg thrust and arm extension (with no leg split) is adequate to elevate a lightweight barbell. With a heavier resistance (which cannot be elevated to arm's length above the head with leg thrust and arm extension alone), the athlete is forced to split the legs at high speed and drop very low under the bar.
10. With the bar held above the head at arm's length, and with the legs split forward and backward, the athlete carefully brings both legs back toward their original position. The athlete finishes the lift standing at attention with the feet shoulder-width apart and with the barbell held at arm's length above the head. This completes an Olympic clean and jerk.	10. With the barbell above the head, the combined center of gravity of athlete and barbell is raised upward, and with increased height, both athlete and barbell become progressively unstable. The athlete must struggle to keep the line of gravity of the barbell centralized above his small, narrow base in order not to lose control and fail in the lift.

Swinging and Rotating Skills

Skill highlights

1. The same mechanical principles that control angular motion govern swinging. In swinging skills an athlete stretches out on the downswing. This action moves the athlete's center of gravity as far from the bar (i.e., the axis of rotation) as possible. By carrying out this action, the athlete allows gravity to exert maximal accelerative torque to his body on the downswing.

2. To rise high on the upswing, an athlete counteracts the decelerating effects of gravity by flexing at the hips and shoulders. This action pulls the athlete's center of gravity closer to the bar, which reduces gravity's decelerative torque.

3. When performing somersaults and other rotary skills on apparatus, or in the air, an eccentric force (i.e., a force that does *not* pass through the athlete's axis of rotation) is applied to the athlete's body at the start of the skill. An eccentric force applies the turning effect of torque to the athlete's body. A slight body lean in the direction of rotation at the instant of takeoff is a common method for applying this eccentric force.

4. Reducing the athlete's rotary resistance during flight increases an athlete's angular velocity (i.e., the athlete's rate of spin). Rotary inertia is reduced by using muscular force to pull the athlete's body mass in toward the axis of rotation. Angular velocity is decreased by extending the athlete's body mass outward from the axis of rotation. This action increases the athlete's rotary inertia and reduces the athlete's rate of spin.

SPOTLIGHT ON . . .

Giant Circle

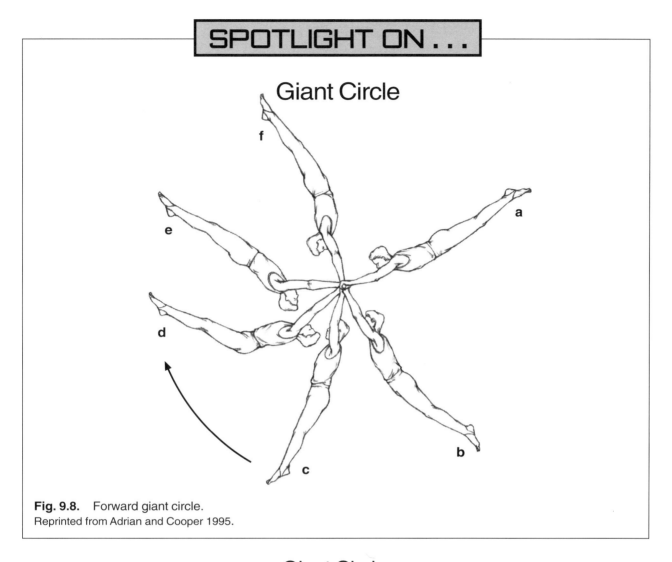

Fig. 9.8. Forward giant circle.
Reprinted from Adrian and Cooper 1995.

Giant Circle

Technique	Mechanics
1. A gymnast frequently begins in a front support position and "casts" (i.e., thrusts against the bar) to elevate his body to a position where his center of gravity is well above the bar.	1. By elevating his center of gravity high above the bar, a gymnast increases his potential energy. Gravity then has the opportunity to accelerate him from greater height on the downswing. The higher a gymnast raises his center of gravity, the greater the time frame during which gravity can accelerate him downward. This increases the athlete's angular velocity and angular momentum.
2. Once well above the bar and beginning the descent, the gymnast stretches to full extension (see Figure 9.8a).	2. By stretching to full extension, a gymnast pushes his center of gravity as far as possible from the axis of rotation (i.e., the bar). This allows gravity to apply the greatest amount of accelerative torque to the gymnast's body on the downswing. Just prior to reaching a position directly below the bar, the gymnast flexes the muscles of the spine. This action prestretches the abdominal muscles ready for flexing the hips when the athlete rises on the upswing (see Figure 9.8b).

Giant Circle

Technique	Mechanics
3. Gravity accelerates the gymnast's body downward.	3. Gravity applies an accelerative torque to the gymnast's body. This torque increases until it is maximal when the gymnast is stretched horizontally from the bar. From that point, although the gymnast's angular velocity and momentum continue to increase, the amount of torque applied to the gymnast's body gets progressively less until it is zero when the gymnast passes directly below the bar.
4. After passing below the bar, the gymnast flexes at the hips and at the shoulders (see Figure 9.8, c-d). Beginners may also flex at the knees.	4. Flexion at the hips and shoulders brings the gymnast's center of gravity closer to the axis of rotation. Gravity's decelerative torque is reduced. By flexing, the gymnast's mass is also pulled closer to the bar. This reduces the gymnast's rotary resistance (i.e., rotary inertia).
5. In a flexed body position a gymnast rises upward. The flexion in the body is progressively eliminated as the athlete moves to a position vertically above the bar (see Figure 9.8, e-f). Some pulling action is applied to the bar to get the gymnast's body over the top of the bar.	5. With a reduction in the gymnast's rotary inertia and a reduction in gravity's decelerative torque, the gymnast is able to rise to a position vertically above his axis of rotation (i.e., the bar). Immediately prior to the vertical position, the athlete can extend in order to slow down (i.e., control) the rate of spin around the bar.
6. Once above the bar and beginning the descent, the gymnast extends the body again to repeat the process described in 1 to 3 above.	6. Above the bar, the gymnast straightens out the body to shift his center of gravity as far from the bar as possible. This allows gravity to reapply maximum torque to the gymnast's body on the downswing. In this way continuous giant circles are performed.

SPOTLIGHT ON . . .

Aerial Front Somersault

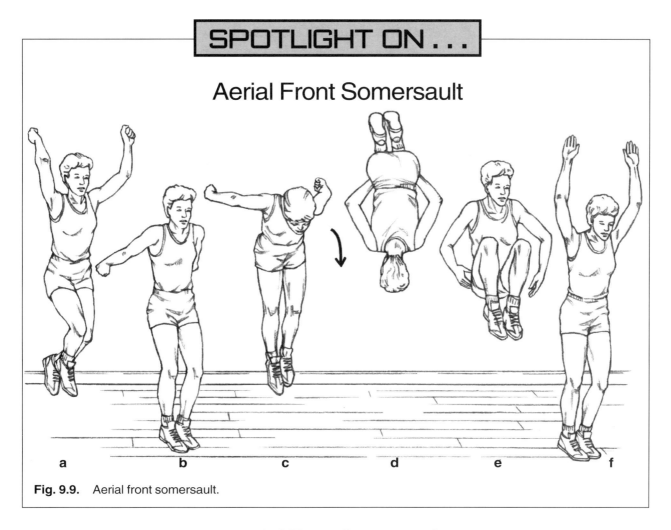

a   b   c   d   e   f

Fig. 9.9. Aerial front somersault.

Aerial Front Somersault

Technique	Mechanics
1. To perform aerial rotations the athlete can begin either with an approach or from standing. An approach allows the athlete to use the same technique as a high jumper for gaining height. The feet are placed ahead of the center of gravity, the quadriceps muscles are prestretched, and the arms are swung upward to assist at takeoff (see Figure 9.9, b-c).	1. An approach before takeoff allows the athlete to position the center of gravity to the rear of the takeoff foot. This allows the athlete to rock forward over the takeoff foot and apply more impulse (force × time) against the takeoff surface. A hurdle-step coupled with a drop onto a sprung surface (e.g., a tumbling mat, beatboard, or trampette) prestretches the quadriceps muscles and stores strain energy in the apparatus. This is added to the athlete's leg thrust to propel the athlete upward.
2. During the takeoff the arms are swung upward at the same time that the legs thrust down at the supporting surface (see Figure 9.9b).	2. Arm swing during the takeoff provides momentum transfer to the athlete's body as a whole. The action of the arms adds to the downward thrust of the legs and increases the reactional force of the takeoff surface (e.g., floor, exercise mat, beatboard, or springboard) thrusting upward against the athlete.

Aerial Front Somersault

Technique	Mechanics
3. The thrust of the legs can be made against a sprung surface (e.g., springboard, beatboard, trampoline, or modern gymnastic floor exercise mat).	3. Downward thrust by the athlete produces flexion in a sprung surface. A sprung surface stores strain energy. The recoil of the flexed surface helps to drive the athlete up in the air.
4. An angle of takeoff close to the vertical, coupled with a powerful upward thrust, guarantees the most airtime for complicated somersaulting (and twisting) skills (see Figure 9.9b). In diving, horizontal movement is necessary to clear the end of the board. This is not the case in floor exercises or during trampoline skills.	4. Vertical thrust is always partially compromised when horizontal movement and rotation are required. To perform the most somersaults in the air, the athlete must thrust downward as close to vertical as possible (to produce the greatest airtime), while still initiating rotation and, in the sport of diving, applying some horizontal thrust to move a safe distance from the board.
5. To initiate rotation, the thrust that drives the athlete upward must not pass through the athlete's center of gravity. Swinging the arms and shifting the head and trunk can assist in promoting rotation (see Figure 9.9, b-c).	5. An eccentric force causing rotation occurs when the upward thrust from the athlete's legs and the supporting surface are directed at a distance from—rather than passing through—the athlete's center of gravity. This produces the turning effect of torque (force × distance from axis of rotation), which causes the athlete to rotate. Rotation can be enhanced when the arms, head, and trunk are also thrown in the direction of rotation. This form of momentum transfer must occur while the athlete is still in contact with the supporting surface.
6. The athlete's flight is set at takeoff and cannot be changed in flight.	6. Any amount of body movement in the air will not change the flight path of the athlete's center of gravity once it is set at takeoff. Likewise an athlete's angular momentum is set at takeoff. Angular momentum at takeoff depends on (a) the mass of the athlete, (b) the distribution of the athlete's mass at takeoff relative to the athlete's axis of rotation, and (c) the angular velocity (i.e., rate of spin) initiated at takeoff.
7. To perform somersaults in the air the athlete must have the following: (a) Vertical thrust to provide optimal airtime (b) A takeoff with the body in an extended position (c) As much rotation at takeoff as possible without compromising airtime or an extended body position (d) Sufficient muscular strength and flexibility to pull the body into the tightest tuck possible while in the air	7. A rotating body in an extended position produces considerable angular momentum. Since angular momentum is conserved in flight, pulling the athlete's body mass inward toward the axis of rotation produces an increase in angular velocity (i.e., rate of spin). A shift from a fully extended body position to the tightest tuck possible results in the greatest increase in the athlete's rate of spin (i.e., angular velocity). In reverse, a shift from a tight tuck to an extended body position reduces the athlete's rate of spin.

Aerial Front Somersault

Technique	Mechanics
8. During flight, axes for somersaults and twists always pass through the athlete's center of gravity.	8. Irrespective of changes in the athlete's body position (i.e., shifting from an extended body position to a tuck), or whatever combination of twist and somersault the athlete performs, axes of rotation always pass through the athlete's center of gravity. Even when apparently out of control, the athlete's body mass is balanced and in a state of equilibrium around the athlete's center of gravity.
9. All actions performed in the air cause equal and opposite reactions to occur. A counterclockwise movement of one part of the athlete's body causes a clockwise movement of some other part. These occur simultaneously. Pulling the head and shoulders forward into a tuck causes the flexed legs to move in the opposing direction, which is toward the head and shoulders (see Figure 9.9, c-d).	9. The arc of movement of the athlete's body segments producing the action and the arc of movement producing the reaction depend on their respective rotary inertia. More massive body segments that are extended farther from the axis of rotation shift a smaller distance (or arc) than those that are less massive and closer to the axis of rotation.
10. Variation of body position in flight allows an athlete to control the number of somersaults (and twists) that are performed. Rotation can be slowed for a head-first entry (in diving) or a feet-first landing (in floor exercises and many skills on the trampoline) (see Figure 9.9, d-f).	10. Compressing the body mass inward toward the axis of rotation reduces its rotary inertia. As angular momentum is conserved in flight, a reduction in rotary inertia causes an increase in angular velocity. Extending the body increases rotary inertia and decreases the athlete's angular velocity.

Equilibrium and Stability

Skill highlights

1. Athletes in the sport of judo and other combative sports use combinations of rotation, pulling, pushing, and lifting to lessen an opponent's stability and set the opponent up for a throw. Opponents counter an attack by leaning toward a push and leaning away from a pull. To increase stability and make themselves less vulnerable, athletes widen their base, and lower and centralize their center of gravity. Weight divisions in combatives are intended to negate advantages gained from body mass.

2. To maintain stability and to destroy the stability of an opponent in judo, and other combative sports, is predominately a battle of one torque versus another. Pushing, pulling, and lifting are used to spin an opponent around axes formed by the athlete's feet, hips, back, and shoulders. Leg sweeps in judo are a common method of eliminating an opponent's base of support.

SPOTLIGHT ON . . .

Judo Hip Throw

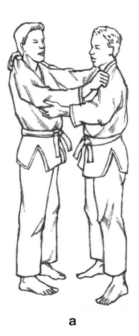   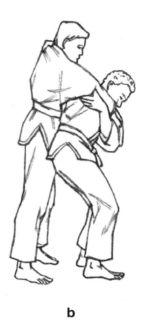

a   b

Fig. 9.10.   Judo hip throw.

Judo Hip Throw

Technique	**Mechanics**
1. Judo involves pushing, pulling, lifting, and rotating, all of which are designed to maintain the attacker's stability while disrupting that of the opponent. Precise timing, coordination, and superfast reactions are essential.	1. The intent of the attacker is to shift the opponent's center of gravity outside of the opponent's supporting base and so destroy his or her stability. Superfast combinations of pushing, pulling, lifting, and rotating are used to achieve this end.
2. Judoka face each other in a standing position with their bodies slightly lowered and with their legs partially flexed. Their feet are at right angles to each other and shoulder-width apart. Fast, shuffling, flat-footed steps are taken with the athlete's body weight frequently positioned closer to the front foot.	2. Lowering the center of gravity increases the stability of the athlete. Positioning the feet at right angles gives good stability side to side and front to back. Fast, shuffling steps increase stability because they limit time spent on one foot. Having the line of the center of gravity closer to the front foot readies the rear leg for leg sweeps and other destabilizing actions used against the opponent.

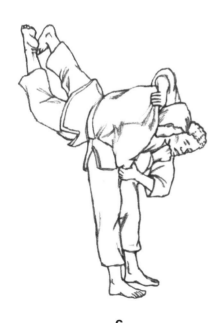

c

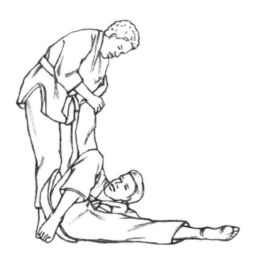

d

Judo Hip Throw

Technique	Mechanics
3. Judoka begin their attacking and defensive maneuvers by grasping each other's tunics on the collar at shoulder level with one hand, and at the sleeve with the other (see Figure 9.10a). Grips are suddenly altered according to the throw being attempted.	3. Grips on the tunic are designed to facilitate push-pull and rotational movements. Any combination can be used. Applying force at the sleeve rotates the opponent around his or her long axis. Applying force at the collar and upper lapel produces forward and backward movement or rotation.
4. With grips on each other's tunics, judoka circle each other waiting for the opportunity to initiate a throw.	4. Preparation for a throw is a series of push-pull rotary actions in which the prime objective is to move the opponent's center of gravity into a position of minimal stability.
5. In a hip throw, which incorporates a lifting action, the attacker grasps the rear part of the right collar with the right hand. The left hand grips the opponent's tunic below the left arm. The attacker pulls the opponent forward with both hands.	5. Pulling the opponent's body forward, the attacker lessens the opponent's stability by moving the line of his center of gravity closer to or beyond the edge of his supporting base. A high grip on the rear collar maximizes the force arm from the collar to the axis of the attacker's hips, over which the opponent will subsequently be rotated. The grip below the left arm will spin (i.e., rotate) the opponent around his long axis.
6. The moment the opponent is successfully drawn forward and destabilized, the attacker quickly initiates a pivot on his left foot by stepping across with his right while flexing the legs (see Figure 9.10b).	6. By rotating his body to the left, the attacker prepares to use his hip as an axis of rotation over which the opponent will be pulled. Flexing his legs, the attacker not only increases his own stability but also prepares to totally destabilize the opponent by lifting him out of contact with the mat (and the earth) when he extends his legs.
7. The attacker's lower back is pressed against the opponent's thighs. The attacker's upper back is pressed against the opponent's stomach. The opponent's upper body is pulled downward over the attacker's hip with both hands while the opponent's feet are lifted off the mat by straightening the attacker's legs (see Figure 9.10c).	7. The attacker's upper hip becomes an axis of rotation over which the opponent rotates. A force is applied by the attacker's hands, which pull (and rotate) the opponent's upper body downward. Another force is applied by the extension of the attacker's legs, which drive the opponent's lower body upward. The opponent spins around the axis of the attacker's hips.

Judo Hip Throw

Technique	Mechanics
8. The opponent's lower body is forced upward taking his feet out of contact with the mat. The opponent's upper body is pulled downward. The opponent rolls over the attacker's hip.	8. The attacker's downward pull and leg extension eliminate the opponent's contact with the mat. Frictional forces between the opponent and the mat no longer exist. The opponent is now defenseless and will be thrown onto his back (see Figure 9.10c).
9. A breakfall is performed by the opponent on contact with the mat (see Figure 9.10d)	9. Totally destabilized, the opponent prepares for the impact with the mat that will occur after the fall. The opponent correctly enlarges the time frame and area over which the impact is made with the mat.

Arresting Motion

Skill highlights

1. Catching, landing, slowing down, and stopping are all forms of arresting motion. Arresting motion involves the forces present in a collision when two or more objects impact together. Athletes need to use correct technique when arresting motion, whether it's their own body, an opponent, or the motion of an inanimate object like a baseball.

2. To safely arrest their own motion, athletes apply a stopping force to their bodies over as large a distance and time frame as possible. In addition, the impact is spread over as big an area as possible. In this way the pressure applied at any one spot to the athlete's body is reduced. Pulling the arm back when catching, flexing the legs and rolling when landing, and using padding and crash pads gradually dissipate the forces that occur during an impact. An athlete can then avoid injury (which occurs when great force is stopped in an instant in a small area) and maintain control and equilibrium when the impact occurs.

SPOTLIGHT ON . . .

Judo Breakfall

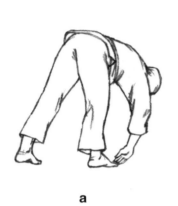 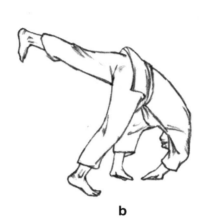 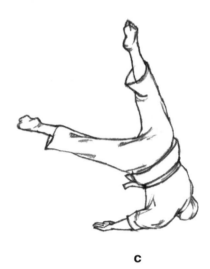

a   b   c

Fig. 9.11. Judo breakfall.

Judo Breakfall

Technique	Mechanics
1. Mastery of ukemi, or the art of falling, is necessary in judo, not only to facilitate movements that follow the fall, but also to prevent injury when a judoka (i.e., a judo practitioner) is thrown.	1. Falls in judo occur from various heights (e.g., from as high as an opponent's shoulders). They also occur at various velocities. The opponent can add his own muscular force to that of gravity. The momentum generated during the fall equals the mass of the falling judoka × his velocity.
2. When a judoka hits the mat, the athlete's velocity is reduced to zero.	2. The judoka's velocity (and momentum) built up during the fall is reduced to zero on contact with the mat. The force with which the judoka hits the mat is applied against the athlete's body by the reaction of the earth.
3. Ukemi teaches the judoka to strike the mat simultaneously with the arms and legs as the trunk makes contact. In this way the trunk is protected because it does not absorb the full force of the fall (see Figure 9.11d).	3. By striking the mat with the arms and legs, the judoka uses the shoulders, thigh, and knee joints as shock absorbers. By carrying out this action, the judoka extends the time frame during which force is applied against the earth and, in reaction from the earth, against the athlete. An extended time frame over which force is applied causes a more gradual change in the judoka's momentum (and kinetic energy), and with it less chance of injury.

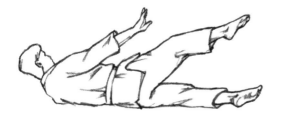
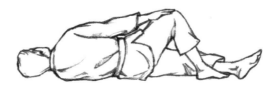

d   e

Judo Breakfall

Technique	Mechanics
4. Judoka attempt to turn vertical movement in a fall into an oblique and subsequently horizontal movement by flexing and bending the body. They roll on the shoulders, back, and on the arm (see Figure 9.11, a-d).	4. A situation where the judoka falls vertically onto the mat brings an athlete to a sudden stop. In this situation, considerable force is applied to the earth, and from the earth against the athlete, in a small time frame. Flexing the legs, squatting down and rolling, extend the time frame during which force is applied by the judoka against the mat, and in reaction by the earth via the mat to the judoka.
5. By rolling and contacting the mat with the extended arm(s) and legs, the judoka enlarges the surface area of the body that contacts the mat (see Figure 9.11, b-e).	5. Enlarging the contact area of the body as the judoka's body contacts the mat decreases the pressure applied at any point of the athlete's body. Enlarging the contact area and extending the time frame that force is applied to the earth (and from the earth to the athlete), significantly reduces the possibility of injury that the athlete might experience from being thrown.

ANSWERS TO QUESTIONS

Chapter 1

1. They study the effects of forces acting on living and nonliving objects.

2. Traditional methods of training have been based for the most part on instinct, copying, and the feeling that if it works for one athlete, it will work for all athletes!

3. An understanding of sport mechanics helps you to accurately assess athletic performance. It also helps you pick out errors in performance accurately (and not haphazardly).

4. Aside from personal idiosyncrasies, the fundamentals of good technique are tied to the physical laws that control our movements on earth, and the same laws apply to athletes. Making the best use of these physical laws produces the similarities you see among athletes performing any skill at an elite level.

5. A basic understanding of the physical laws controlling our movement on earth—and how these laws relate to sport techniques—will enable you to make an accurate (rather than a haphazard) assessment of any new method of performing a sport skill.

6. An efficient technique has an appearance of smoothness and coordination, and an efficient use of power.

Chapter 2

1. Yes, weight is a function of the attractive force of gravity. The closer an athlete is to the earth's core, the greater the pull of gravity is and the more the athlete weighs. The earth is not perfectly round, and an athlete is closer to the center of the earth standing at the North or South Pole than standing at the equator. Height above sea level is also a factor, so an athlete standing at the top of a mountain at the equator reduces the effect of gravity even more. At the equator not only will an athlete be farther from the earth's core, but, because of the extra distance from the earth's axis as the earth spins around, the athlete's mass pulls away more from the earth than when he stands either at the North or South Pole. A very sensitive scale could register the difference.

2. The earth and the shot pull on each other with the same force. The earth moves toward the shot, relative to its mass. The earth's tremendous mass gives it a phenomenal amount of inertia, so it moves an immeasurably small distance toward the shot. The shot, having little mass and inertia, does most of the moving, so it accelerates toward the earth.

3. An athlete (e.g., a springboard diver) gains an additional velocity of 32 ft/sec with every second that he falls toward the water. Gravity's acceleration adds a velocity of 32 ft/sec for every second of fall (i.e., 32 ft/sec/sec or 32 ft/sec^2). If we wrote 32 ft/sec (with one distance unit and one time unit), it would indicate velocity but not acceleration. In the metric system, an athlete picks up an additional 9.8 m/sec for every second that he falls toward the water.

4. When a skier extends her legs, she presses down against the earth, and the earth reacts by pushing upward with an equal and

opposite force. This increases the friction between the skis and the snow. By flexing her legs, the skier momentarily reduces the pressure of her body against the earth. The earth, in response, reduces its reaction force. The reduction in these forces decreases the friction between the skis and the snow. Weighting (extension) and unweighting (flexion) assist in carving turns and in other skiing maneuvers.

5. Lean, lightweight athletes tend to have a better strength to weight ratio than more massive athletes. Having less mass, squash and badminton players also have less inertia to fight against than do more massive athletes, so they can stop, start, and maneuver more easily.

6. The quarterback assesses the velocity of the receiver cutting across the field. He also assesses the distance from where he is throwing the ball to the place where the ball will be received. The quarterback then applies the right amount of force in a vertical and horizontal direction (taking into account environmental forces, such as the force of the wind and its direction). The ball must also be spun to better maintain its trajectory.

Chapter 3

1. The answer is the collective mass of the goalkeeper plus the ball. They form a single large mass and accelerate backward into the goal.

2. The baseball is traveling at tremendous velocity and has phenomenal momentum. The forces exerted by the ball on your hand (when you don't pull your arm back) are reduced to zero in an instant. It is your hand reducing this great force over a minimal time frame that causes so much pain! When you wear a glove, it helps extend the time frame over which the ball's momentum is reduced to zero. The glove also spreads the pressure exerted by the ball over a larger area than if you used your hand alone. Drawing your arm back at the instant of contact lengthens the time frame that the momentum of the ball is reduced to zero, lessening the force (or pressure) that the ball exerts on your hand at any instant during the catching sequence.

3. A ball given topspin will arc downward toward the ground more vigorously than a ball given no spin. The topspin applies a Magnus force (i.e., a Magnus effect) that acts toward the surface of the earth. The Magnus force is assisted by gravity's downward pull, giving the ball its tight arc toward the earth. A ball given backspin has a Magnus force acting in opposition to gravity. A powerful backspin causes the ball to lift upward. As the spin dies, the Magnus force weakens and counteracts to a lesser degree the downward pull of gravity.

4. The athlete has finished traveling upward and is no longer moving, so his kinetic energy is zero. Because he's at the top of his flight path, his potential energy is maximum. The pole, having done its job and straightened out because the athlete is at the peak of the vault, has zero strain energy. The force of gravity still exists, even though for an instant the athlete feels weightless and is traveling neither upward or downward.

5. The distance the sled slides is an expression of work performed by an object that has motion. The energy that an object possesses by virtue of its motion is called kinetic energy. If you double the velocity of a moving object, you square its kinetic energy. On the second run the sled has four times the kinetic energy and four times the ability to do work. Consequently the sled will slide about four times farther.

6. The mass of the athlete's body in a one-handed handstand is supported by a much smaller base than in a two-handed handstand. If the gymnast could balance on the tip of a single finger, rather than on one hand, the pressure on the finger would be even greater because the supporting base has been reduced even more!

Chapter 4

1. The distance between the insertion of the biceps on the forearm and the elbow joint (i.e., the axis of rotation) is virtually the same for athletes of the same age and maturity. What varies greatly is the length of athletes' forearms. A long forearm lengthens the size of the resistance arm, and thus it increases the resistive torque produced by the dumbbell. Consequently, an athlete with long forearms must produce more muscular force than an athlete with short forearms.

2. By holding the bat at the hitting end you have shifted the mass of the bat closer to the axis around which you are swinging it. Mass that is shifted closer to the axis of rotation reduces rotary inertia. Consequently, it is easier to accelerate, decelerate, and maneuver the bat when you hold it at the barrel end. Of course, this does not mean that you will hit a baseball farther when holding the bat in this fashion!

3. When you swing your arms upward at takeoff, the swing's momentum is transferred to your body as a whole. The arm swing combines with your leg thrust downward against the earth. In reaction, the earth thrusts upward with greater force. Adding the arm swing to the leg thrust means the earth returns more thrust to the athlete.

4. An athlete's angular momentum is the product of three components: the athlete's rate of spin (i.e., angular velocity), the athlete's mass, and the distribution of the athlete's mass (i.e., how extended or compressed the athlete is relative to his axis of rotation). The flight of athletes in the events mentioned lasts only a very short time. The athletes cannot push or pull against the air to increase or decrease their angular momentum. As a result, the angular momentum that they give themselves at takeoff stays the same (i.e., it is conserved) for the duration of the flight.

5. The athlete's hips lift upward. Timed correctly, this reaction helps the athlete clear the bar.

6. The cat twist and the hula hoop twist.

Chapter 5

1. With your body pressed against the wall, you will find that a toe-touch action pushes your center of gravity ahead (in front) of your toes, which is the perimeter of your base. You topple forward. The same action performed away from the wall allows you to keep your center of gravity within your supporting base as you lean forward: you maintain your balance and do not topple forward.

2. The athlete's foot on the beam is an important axis of rotation. If the athlete tips to one side, gravity provides the force; the distance of the athlete's line of gravity from the axis of rotation provides the other component of a destabilizing torque. The athlete must use muscular force to produce a torque that will counteract this destabilizing torque.

3. Assume that the attacker pushes against the defender from the left and continues to push against the defender from left to right. If the defender enlarges his base from right to left, then more torque is required to destabilize him than if his base was not enlarged. In this situation the defender will usually shift his center of gravity toward the left as well.

4. Maximal stability means widening the base, lowering the center of gravity, and shifting the line of gravity into the center. Such a position would mean that far too much time is taken shifting the athlete's line of gravity toward the perimeter of his supporting base when the athlete is required to move quickly in a particular direction. It is better if the athlete's base is reduced in size and the legs are partially flexed, ready to drive quickly in whatever direction is necessary.

5. The heavier the discus, the faster it spins, and the farther its mass is distributed from its axis of rotation, the better it can fight against external forces that would disturb its flight.

6. When a weight lifter weighing 200 lb raises twice his body weight to arm's length above his head he is elevating the combined center of gravity of himself and the barbell vertically a considerable distance. Raising the mass of any object above the surface of the earth reduces its stability. The weight lifter's feet are close together: This position decreases the size of the weight lifter's supporting base. The slightest movement of the barbell is likely to destabilize the weight lifter.

Chapter 6

1. When a diver breathes compressed air from a scuba tank at any depth, the diver is breathing air at the same pressure as the water at that depth. At a depth of 66 ft the pressure is triple that on the surface and this pressure exists in the lungs. If the diver holds his breath at 66 ft and ascends to the surface, the pressure in the lungs is reduced to one third and the air in the lungs triples in volume! Serious injury or death can occur from this action.

2. Fat weighs less per unit of volume than do bone and muscle. The sumo wrestler will occupy an immense space in the water and, in return, will likely experience a buoyant force greater than his weight of 400 lb. The lean, muscular gymnast will likely experience a buoyant force less than 100 lb, and, as a result, he will sink.

3. John was pulled along in the low suction wake of the pace vehicle. In this position, streamlining was unnecessary.

4. Drag forces are reduced dramatically when cycling in a recumbent position and when a cyclist is enveloped in an aerodynamic shell. The top speed by a sprint cyclist is about 45 mph. Athletes cycling in a recumbent position, and totally covered with an aerodynamic shell, have reached speeds close to 70 mph.

5. The air flowing over the curved upper side of an airfoil is forced to accelerate. The air flowing past the flat underside of the airfoil experiences no change in velocity. Bernoulli's principle states that a fluid (e.g., air) that is forced to accelerate exerts less pressure than the same fluid traveling slower. There is less pressure above the curved side of the wing than below it, and the pressure differential causes a lift force to occur.

6. A spinning ball drags around with it a boundary layer of air. On one side the boundary layer collides with the air passing by. Airflow is decelerated at this point, and a high pressure zone is set up. On the opposing side, the boundary layer is moving in the same direction as the air passing by, so there is no collision and the air collectively moves faster. As a result a low-pressure area is set up. The pressure differential, high on one side and low on the other, creates a lift force causing the ball to move in the direction of the pressure differential (i.e., from high to low).

Chapter 7

1. The objectives and the special characteristics of the skill ultimately determine what technique is used in a skill. If you do not fully understand a skill's objectives and characteristics, you may recommend a technique that satisfies one objective of the skill but does not satisfy other important objectives.

2. A predictable environment is a situation in which an athlete can perform a skill without expecting sudden changes in weather or field conditions and without having to face and counteract the maneuvers of an opponent. Two examples are weight lifting and a synchronized swimming routine.

3. No two athletes are exactly alike. A young, immature athlete will not have the power, coordination, or endurance of an elite athlete. Modifications must be made, but the *basics* of a technique used by elite athletes can be taught to the young as the foundation of skilled performance.

4. The process of analysis is made easier when a skill is divided into phases. It lessens the possibility of confusion that can occur when you try to analyze all of the complex movements of a complete skill simultaneously.

5. A skill can be viewed as a building: The phases are the building's walls, and the key elements are the bricks in the walls. Breaking down a skill into phases and key elements helps in its analysis and in the correction of errors.

6. Each element in each phase of a skill serves a particular mechanical purpose. If you do not know the mechanical reasons for performing each key element in a particular way, you likely will allow any manner of performance, being unable to discern why one action is better than another.

Chapter 8

1. Begin by observing the whole performance and assessing its results. Then shift your attention to the preliminary movements and mental set. Progress to the windup (or recovery) and to the force-producing phase and follow-through. This sequence is good because errors in earlier phases influence the phases that follow.

2. The recovery in a swimming stroke sets the athlete up for a repeat of the force-producing phase. The follow-through in a throwing skill does not set the athlete up for a repeat of the skill but rather works to dissipate the energy of the force-producing action.

3. Usually there is an appearance of tension, stiffness, and poor coordination. The athlete

appears tight, and the performance appears awkward and jerky. In throwing and hitting skills novices commonly apply force with the muscles that move smaller body segments before the larger muscle groups have accelerated the athlete's body as a whole, and, immediately thereafter, they move the larger, heavier body segments. In throwing skills this incorrect sequence gives the appearance of the athlete throwing with the arm alone and forgetting to use the rest of the body!

4. Too much or too little muscular force over too long or too short a time frame produces less than an optimal performance. Superior coaches talk of "timing" and "coordination" when they coach a skill. They also say, "Easy at the start" and "Fast at the finish" or "Float through this section" and "Explode at the finish." Such commands teach athletes to apply the right amount of force for the proper duration.

5. A major error is any factor that seriously detracts from an athlete's ability to apply force optimally. Poor balance, poor timing, and incorrect application of force in amount, timing, and direction are all major errors in the performance of a skill.

6. You can refer to texts on your chosen sport that offer successful teaching methods and techniques for the correction of errors. You can attend coaching seminars and workshops where you can gain information from experienced coaches and specialists in the field. You can make use of information gained from research using the most up-to-date video and computer technology.

GLOSSARY

acceleration—The rate of change of velocity. An athlete can accelerate, decelerate, or have zero acceleration. In the latter case, the athlete is either motionless or moving at a uniform rate.

angle of attack—The angle between the long axis of an object (e.g., a javelin) or an athlete and the direction of fluid (e.g., air) flowing past: on a discus, the angle by which the leading edge is raised or lowered relative to the air flow passing over the implement.

angle of projection—The angle relative to the horizontal at which an object (e.g., a baseball) is projected (e.g., thrown): for example, the angle relative to the horizontal when the athlete takes off in events like the high jump, long jump, and diving.

angular momentum—The quantity of motion that a rotating, spinning, or turning athlete or object possesses. In mechanical terms the angular momentum of any object is determined by the product of the object's mass × the distribution of its mass × its angular velocity.

angular motion—Motion that is circular or rotary, such as somersaulting, twisting, rolling, swinging, rocking, spiraling, and pirouetting.

angular velocity—The rate of spin of an athlete or object. This takes into consideration the number of revolutions, the time frame, and the direction of rotation.

apex—The highest point in a trajectory: for example, in a dive the topmost point of the athlete's flight path.

Archimedes' principle—Named after Archimedes, a Greek mathematician, the principle that the buoyant force acting on an object is equal to the weight of the fluid that the object displaces. If a swimmer weighs more than the weight of the water she displaces when immersed, the athlete will sink. Conversely, if a swimmer weighs less than the weight of the displaced water, she will float.

attitude angle—The angle formed between the horizontal and the long axis of an object. When a discus or a javelin travels through the air its position in the air changes continuously, causing its attitude angle to change. When an athlete releases a discus, its attitude angle and release angle are often the same.

axis of rotation—An imaginary line that passes through the center of rotation of an object or an athlete. When an athlete or object rotates in flight, the axis of rotation passes through the center of gravity. In contact with the ground, however, the axis of rotation and center of gravity are often in different positions.

balance—The ability of an athlete to maintain or control a state of equilibrium.

base of support—The area formed by the outermost points of contact between an object or athlete and their supporting surfaces. The base of support is not necessarily beneath the object.

Bernoulli's principle—Named after Daniel Bernoulli, a Swiss mathematician, the principle states that pressure exerted by a fluid is inversely proportional to its velocity. Fluids (e.g., air and water) exert less pressure the faster they move; conversely, fluids exert more pressure the slower they move.

biomechanics—The application of the laws and principles of mechanics to living organisms.

body tilt twist—Technique that divers use in which they tilt the body away from its somersaulting axis, causing some of their angular momentum to go into the twisting axis and allowing them to twist and somersault simultaneously.

boundary layer—The layer of fluid contacting the surface of an object or an athlete immersed or moving in a fluid. Swimmers can have a boundary layer of air passing over those parts of their bodies moving through the air or of water for those parts moving through the water.

buoyancy—A force in fluids that lifts upward and fights against gravity: A buoyant force occurs both in water and in air. It is greater in water than in air because of water's greater density.

buoyant force—An upward force opposing gravity, exerted on an immersed object by the fluid beneath it. See Archimedes' principle.

cat twist—A diving technique imitating a cat falling to the ground and landing on all four feet. This involves bending at the hips and twisting, turning one part of the body with less rotary inertia against another part with more rotary inertia.

center of buoyancy—A point at which the buoyant force acts on an immersed object. For an athlete the center of buoyancy is commonly higher on the body than the center of gravity.

center of gravity—A point at which the mass and weight of an object or an athlete are balanced in all directions. It is also that point where gravitational forces are centralized. The center of gravity for males is usually higher than for females.

centrifugal force—Centrifugal force is, in reality, inertia—whose tendency is to keep rotating objects moving in a straight line rather than around a circular pathway.

centripetal force—A force that acts radially inward toward the axis of rotation of a rotating object and that is responsible for holding the object to its rotary path.

closed skills—Skills that are performed in a predictable, controlled environment. Synchronized swimming is an example of a closed skill.

conservation of angular momentum—Having a set amount of angular momentum remain for the duration of an action. An object or athlete will continue to rotate with constant angular momentum unless an external torque increases or decreases its angular momentum. During the flight from the tower to the water, a diver has virtually the same amount of angular momentum from takeoff until contact with the water.

conservation of energy—The law stating that the amount of energy in the universe is constant and cannot be created or destroyed—only changed in form. When an athlete slows down and gives up kinetic energy, his energy is transformed into other forms, such as heat, movement, and distortion of whatever the athlete contacts. The total amount of energy remains unchanged.

density—Weight or mass per unit volume: the amount of substance contained in a particular space. The greater the amount, the greater the density. An athlete's muscles and bones are more dense than fat.

drag—A force produced by the relative motion of an object or an athlete in a fluid (e.g., water or air). The direction that drag force acts is in opposition to the motion of the object or athlete through the fluid.

elasticity—The ability of an object to recover its original shape after being deformed. Golf balls, archery bows, and modern composite vaulting poles are all highly elastic.

equilibrium—A state in which there is neither acceleration nor deceleration. Athletes seldom exhibit an absolute state of equilibrium. Elite athletes performing handstands still exhibit some motion, and thus are continuously accelerating and decelerating.

first class lever—A lever in which the axis is positioned in seesaw fashion between the force and the resistance. If the force arm is longer than the resistance arm, a first class lever favors force. If the resistance arm is longer than the force arm, the first class lever favors speed and range of movement at the expense of force.

flexibility—The range of motion in an athlete's joints. Flexibility is also used to describe the flex of an object (e.g., vaulting pole).

follow-through (or recovery)—The actions that occur as soon as the force-producing movements are completed. Usually the athlete, or her limbs, continue along the original pathway because of momentum. A follow-through safely dissipates the force of the actions.

force—Any influence that tends to change the state of motion of an object or its dimensions. Force applied by an athlete does not necessarily have to produce movement.

force arm—The perpendicular distance from where the force acts on a lever to the axis of rotation.

force-producing movements—The specific actions an athlete uses to generate force in a skill.

force vectors—The combination of the direction of force and the amount of applied force. In mechanics, force vector is diagrammatically represented by an arrow.

form drag—Drag caused by the shape of an object moving through a fluid (also called *profile drag*, *pressure drag*, and *shape drag*). When an athlete (or an object) travels through a fluid, high pressure occurs in front, where the athlete contacts the fluid head on, and low pressure occurs immediately to the rear of the athlete: The greater the difference between high and low pressure, the greater the form drag.

friction—A force that acts in opposition to the movement of one surface on another. The various types of friction include static, sliding, and rolling friction.

fulcrum—An axis or hinge about which a lever rotates.

gravitational acceleration—The rate of acceleration of an object or athlete toward the earth, commonly stated as 32 ft/sec^2 (or 9.8 m/sec^2).

gravity—The force that attracts an object or an athlete to the center of the earth. Gravitational forces also exist on other celestial bodies.

ground reaction force—The equal and opposite force exerted by the earth in response to a force exerted against the earth. An athlete pressing against the earth with a certain force causes the earth to respond both equally and in the opposite direction with a force of the same magnitude.

horsepower—A term used by inventor James Watt when comparing the output of a steam engine to that of a horse performing the same work. One horsepower is the ability of an object or an athlete to move 550 lb a distance of 1 ft in a time frame of 1 sec. One horsepower is the equivalent of 746 watts in the metric system.

hula hoop twist—A twisting technique used by divers and gymnasts during flight in which the hips are rotated, causing the upper and lower body to rotate in one direction and the body as a whole to rotate in the opposite direction.

hydrostatic pressure—The pressure (i.e., force/area) exerted by a fluid (e.g., air or water) to support its own weight or the weight of an object or an athlete immersed in the fluid. Atmospheric pressure is 14.7 lb per square inch at sea level. Sea water exerts a pressure of 14.7 lb per square inch for every 33 ft of depth.

impact—A collision between two or more objects.

impulse—The product of force multiplied by the time during which the force acts. Athletes vary the amount of muscular force and the time frame over which their force is applied.

inertia—The tendency of an object or athlete to either stay at rest or to move continuously in a straight line at a uniform velocity. Inertia is directly related to mass. A more massive athlete or object has greater inertia than one with less mass. (See Newton's First Law.)

key elements—Distinct actions that together make up a phase: These vary for each phase of a skill.

kinetic energy—The ability of an object or athlete to perform work by virtue of their motion. Doubling the mass of a moving object increases its kinetic energy twofold; doubling the velocity of a moving object increases its kinetic energy fourfold.

kinetic friction—The friction generated between two surfaces that are sliding, or moving, against each other.

laminar flow—A flow pattern in fluids characterized by smooth, parallel lines (e.g., laminations in wood). Laminar flow occurs when fluids pass objects and athletes at very low velocities.

lever—A simple mechanism consisting of a relatively rigid bar-like object rotating about an axis. The body's bones, joints, and muscles work together as lever systems.

lift—The force acting on an object in a fluid, perpendicular to the fluid's flow. Lift is not always upward: It can occur in any direction.

linear motion—All parts of an athlete or object moving in the same direction at the same speed. Also called *translation*.

linear stability—An athlete's or object's resistance against being moved in a certain direction; resistance against being stopped or forced to change direction once moving.

line of gravity—An invisible vertical line passing through an athlete's or an object's center of gravity.

longitudinal axis—An imaginary line that runs the length of an object; also called the long axis.

Magnus effect—Named after Gustav Magnus, a German scientist; the movement of the trajectory of a spinning object (such as a baseball or soccer ball) toward the direction of spin. If the front or leading surface of a baseball is spinning to the left, for example, the Magnus effect causes the flight path to bend to the left.

Magnus force—A lift force created by the spin of an object (such as a baseball, soccer ball, or golfball); see Magnus effect.

mass—The amount of matter, or substance, in an object. A massive athlete has considerable body mass. Mass is also a measure of an object's or athlete's inertia. A more massive athlete has more inertia than a less massive athlete.

matter—Anything having weight on the surface of the earth and occupying space. Matter has mass and inertia.

meter—A unit of length based on the metric system. One meter equals 3.281 ft. The 1500 m race in the Olympics is 120 yd short of a mile.

moment of inertia—The same as rotary inertia or rotary resistance. Rotary inertia varies according to the mass of a rotating object and the distance that its mass is distributed, relative to its axis of rotation. An athlete has greater rotary inertia somersaulting in an extended body position than in a tight tuck.

momentum—Quantity of motion; the mass of an object multiplied by its velocity. Increase the mass or the velocity, and you increase momentum.

negative acceleration—A decrease in velocity of a moving object or an athlete.

newton—A measurement used in the metric system and named in honor of Sir Isaac Newton's contributions to science. Applied to a mass of one kilogram, a newton is a force that gives it an acceleration of 1 m/sec^2. A newton = .2248 lb.

Newton's First Law (the law of inertia)—All athletes and objects have mass and, thus, inertia. Their inertia is expressed by a desire to remain at rest. If a force is applied to get them moving, their inertia gives them the tendency to travel at the same velocity in a straight line. (Forces applied by gravity, friction, air resistance, etc. naturally alter this state.)

Newton's Second Law (the law of acceleration)—The acceleration of an object or an athlete is proportional to the force acting on it, and inversely proportional to its mass. A massive athlete accelerates less in the direction that force is applied than does a less massive athlete.

Newton's Third Law (the law of action and reaction)—When an object or athlete exerts a force on a second object (or athlete), the latter exerts a reaction force on the first, which is both equal and opposite in direction.

nonrepetitive skills—Often called discrete skills; skills that have a definite beginning and finish and that do not repeat in a cyclic fashion. Examples are a hip throw in judo and a slap shot in ice hockey.

open skills—Skills performed in an unpredictable environment, the unpredictability coming from the opposition or the environment.

phase—A connected group of movements that seemingly "stand on their own" but that join together in the performance of the total skill.

positive acceleration—An increase in velocity of a moving object or athlete.

potential energy—The ability to do work by virtue of height above the earth's surface. Potential energy increases as you increase the height and/or the mass of an athlete or an object situated above the surface of the earth.

power—The rate at which mechanical work is done (i.e., force multiplied by the distance that the resistance is moved). Power is work divided by the time taken to perform the work.

pressure—Force per unit area. Pressure is the ratio of force to the area over which force is applied. The same force applied over a larger area exerts less pressure per unit of area.

projectiles—Objects that are propelled into the air. Athletes themselves can also be projectiles.

propulsive drag—Drag force acting in the same direction as an object or athlete is traveling.

radial distribution of mass—The mass of an object and how it is distributed (or positioned) relative to its axis of rotation.

rebound—The action of objects separating or moving away from one another after an impact or collision.

relative motion—The motion of one item relative to another.

repetitive skills—Often called non-discrete skills. These are skills that are continuous, repetitious, and cyclic in motion (e.g., swimming, cycling, and cross-country skiing).

resistance—Anything that provides an opposing force (e.g., the athlete's body plus whatever object the athlete is holding, pushing, throwing).

resistance arm—The perpendicular distance from where the resistance acts on a lever to the axis of rotation.

resultant force vector—A single vector that results from the combination of several vectors. Several forces acting in unison on an object can produce a single equivalent force: The direction and amount of the resulting force is called a resultant force vector.

rotary inertia—The tendency of objects to initially resist rotation and then to continue rotating once started.

rotary stability—An athlete's or object's resistance against being tilted or rotated in some way. Once rotating, it is the ability to continue rotating.

scalar measurement—A quantity that gives magnitude but not direction: 20 mph is a scalar measurement indicating only speed. (Velocity indicates both speed and direction.)

second class lever—A lever in which the resistance is positioned between the axis and the force. Second class levers favor force rather than speed and distance.

skill—A movement pattern designed to satisfy the demands of a sport or a specific activity.

skill objectives—Objectives determined by the rules of the sport and the conditions under which a skill is performed. These objectives determine the techniques and mechanics the athlete must use to perform the skill successfully.

speed—An athlete's or an object's movement per unit of time, with no consideration to direction.

stability—Resistance to the disturbance of equilibrium.

strain energy—A form of potential energy stored in an object when it is distorted or deformed. An archer's bow and a vaulter's pole store strain energy.

strength—The ability of a muscle (or muscles) to exert force against a resistance (without consideration of the time that force is applied).

style—Personal variations an athlete makes to a skill, technique, or pattern of movements.

surface drag—Also called skin drag, viscous drag, and skin friction; the drag that occurs moves when a fluid (e.g., air or water) contacts the surfaces of an object or an athlete that is moving through the fluid.

technique—A commonly used method by which a skill is performed.

third class lever—A lever in which the applied force is positioned between the axis and the resistance. Third class levers, which favor the magnification of speed and distance at the expense of force, are the most common lever systems in the human body.

torque—A rotary, turning, or twisting effect produced by a force acting at a distance from the axis of rotation. The initiation of rotation requires the application of torque.

trajectory—The aerial pathway followed by an object or athlete.

translation—A term for linear motion.

turbulent flow—A disturbed flow pattern in a fluid.

uniform acceleration—Acceleration that is regular, occurring when velocity increases at a regular rate.

uniform deceleration—Deceleration that is regular, occurring when velocity decreases at a regular rate.

velocity—The speed of an athlete or object in a given direction. Velocity can change when direction changes, even though speed may remain uniform.

viscosity—A measure of fluid's "stickiness" and resistance to flow. An increase in water temperature decreases its viscosity. An increase in air temperature slightly increases its viscosity.

volume—The amount of space occupied by an object or athlete.

vortex—A mass of swirling liquid. Swimmers use vortexes to help cancel drag and assist in propulsion.

wake—An area of turbulence, consisting of swirling low pressure and suction, that occurs behind an object or athlete traveling at high speed.

wave drag—The drag created by the action of waves at the interface between two fluids. In sport, wave drag occurs where air and water meet.

weight—The force on an object or athlete exerted by the earth's attraction.

windup (or backswing)—A movement that stretches the athlete's muscles and establishes a position from which he can apply force over a long distance or time frame.

work—In mechanics work is force multiplied by the distance through which a resistance is moved. A diver climbing the steps of the tower performs work because the diver's mass is raised a certain distance. No mechanical work is performed in isometric exercises because an athlete applies force against an object without causing movement.

BIBLIOGRAPHY

Adrian, M.J., & Cooper, J.M. (1989). *Biomechanics of Human Movement*. Indianapolis: Benchmark.

Blanding, S.L., & Monteleone, J.M. (1992). *What Makes a Boomerang Come Back: The Science of Sports*. Stamford, CT: Longmeadow.

Brancazio, P.J. (1984). *Sport Science: Physical Laws and Optimum Performance*. New York: Simon & Schuster.

Christina, R.W., & Corcos, D.M. (1988). *Coaches Guide to Teaching Sport Skills*. American Coaching Effectiveness Program. Level 2 Sport Science Curriculum. Champaign, IL: Human Kinetics.

Coaching Association of Canada. (1988). *National Coaching Certification Program. Theory Levels 1-5*. Ottawa, ON: Coaching Association of Canada.

Diagram Group. (1982). *The Sports Fan's Ultimate Book of Sports Comparisons*. New York: St. Martins.

Dyson, G. (1986). *Mechanics of Athletics* (8th ed.). Kent, England: Hodder and Stoughton.

Ecker, T. (1971). *Track and Field Dynamics*. Los Altos, CA: TAFNEWS.

Epstein, L.C., (1988). *Thinking Physics: Practical Lessons in Critical Thinking*. San Francisco: Insight.

Griffing, D.F. (1984). *The Dynamics of Sports: Why That's the Way the Ball Bounces*. Oxford, OH: Dialog.

Hall, S.J. (1991). *Basic Biomechanics*. St. Louis, MO: Mosby.

Hay, J.G. (1993). *The Biomechanics of Sports Techniques* (4th ed.). Englewood Cliffs, NJ: Prentice Hall.

Hay, J.G., & Reid, G.J. (1988). *Anatomy, Mechanics, and Human Motion*. Englewood Cliffs, NJ: Prentice Hall.

Kreighbaum, E., & Barthels, K.M. (1990). *Biomechanics. A Qualitative Approach For Studying Human Movement* (3rd ed.). New York: Macmillan.

Maglischo, E.W. (1982). *Swimming Faster*. Palo Alto, CA: Mayfield.

Matthews, P. (Ed.) (1993). *The Guinness Book of Records 1993*. New York: Bantam.

Pearl, B. (1980). *Bill Pearl's Keys to the Inner Universe: Encyclopedia on Weight Training*. Pasadena, CA: Typecraft.

Pearl, B., & Moran, G.T. (1986). *Getting Stronger*. Bolinas, CA: Shelter.

Schultz, R. (1992). *Looking Inside Sports Aerodynamics*. Santa Fe, NM: John Muir.

Sports Illustrated. (1993). 1993 Sports Almanac. Boston: Little, Brown.

Walker, J. (1977). *The Flying Circus of Physics—With Answers*. New York: Wiley.

Wallechinsky, D. (1991). *The Complete Book of the Olympics. 1992 Edition*. Boston: Little, Brown.

INDEX

ABOUT THE AUTHOR

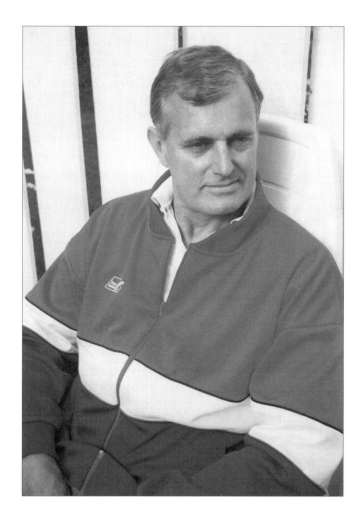

Gerry Carr, professor of physical education at the University of Victoria, British Columbia, Canada, also teaches sport mechanics to coaches at the National Coaching Institute at the University of Victoria. In his university courses, Dr. Carr found that students responded better when he de-emphasized calculations, teaching relationships and concepts rather than formulas. That approach forms the basis of this book.

Dr. Carr is a member of many professional organizations, including the Canadian Coaching Association and the Canadian Society for the History of Sport and Physical Education. He publishes extensively in the area of sport history and sport and politics. Dr. Carr has also written numerous books and articles on teaching and safety in gymnastics and on the fundamentals of track and field.

As a student, Dr. Carr competed for Britain in the Olympics as a discus thrower and earned a scholarship to UCLA, where he represented the Bruins in the throwing events.

Dr. Carr earned his PhD from the University of Stellenbosch, South Africa, in 1974.

American Sport Education Program
Higher Education for Coaches

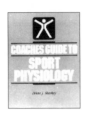

Coaches Guide to Sport Physiology

Brian J. Sharkey, PhD

Coaches Guide
1986 • Paper • 240 pp • Item BSHA0038
ISBN 0-931250-38-2 • $22.00 ($32.95 Canadian)
Study Guide
1986 • Three-Ring Notebook • 276 pp
Item ACEP0202 • ISBN 0-87322-061-7
$32.00 ($47.95 Canadian)

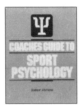

Coaches Guide to Sport Psychology

Rainer Martens, PhD

Coaches Guide
1987 • Paper • 208 pp • Item BMAR0022
ISBN 0-87322-022-6 • $22.00 ($32.95 Canadian)
Study Guide
1989 • Three-Ring Notebook • 432 pp
Item ACEP0204 • ISBN 0-87322-023-4
$32.00 ($47.95 Canadian)

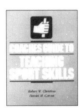

Coaches Guide to Teaching Sport Skills

**Robert W. Christina, PhD, and
Daniel M. Corcos, PhD**

Coaches Guide
1988 • Paper • 168 pp • Item BCHR0020
ISBN 0-87322-020-X • $22.00 ($32.95 Canadian)
Study Guide
1989 • Three-Ring Notebook • 224 pp
Item ACEP0205 • ISBN 0-87322-021-8
$32.00 ($47.95 Canadian)

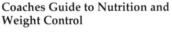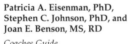

Coaches Guide to Nutrition and Weight Control

(Second Edition)

**Patricia A. Eisenman, PhD,
Stephen C. Johnson, PhD, and
Joan E. Benson, MS, RD**

Coaches Guide
1990 • Paper • 192 pp • Item PEIS0365
ISBN 0-88011-365-0 • $22.00 ($32.95 Canadian)
Study Guide
1991 • Comb-Bound • 208 pp
Item ACEP0207 • ISBN 0-88011-385-5
$32.00 ($47.95 Canadian)

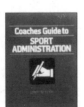

Coaches Guide to Sport Administration

Larry M. Leith, PhD

Coaches Guide
1990 • Paper • 96 pp • Item PLEI0379
ISBN 0-88011-379-0 • $18.00 ($26.95 Canadian)
Study Guide
1990 • Comb-Bound • 136 pp • Item ACEP0206
ISBN 0-88011-382-0 • $26.00 ($38.95 Canadian)

Coaches Guide to Sport Law

**Gary Nygaard, PhD, and
Thomas H. Boone, JD**

Coaches Guide
1985 • Paper • 120 pp
Item BNYG0094 • ISBN 0-931250-94-3
$18.00 ($26.95 Canadian)
Study Guide
1985 • Three-Ring Notebook • 240 pp
Item ACEP0200 • ISBN 0-931250-95-1
$26.00 ($38.95 Canadian)

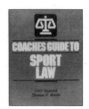

Coaches Guide to Time Management

Charles E. Kozoll, PhD

Coaches Guide
1985 • Paper • 152 pp
Item BKOZ0097 • ISBN 0-931250-97-8
$18.00 ($26.95 Canadian)
Study Guide
1985 • Three-Ring Notebook • 144 pp
Item ACEP0201 • ISBN 0-931250-98-6
$26.00 ($38.95 Canadian)

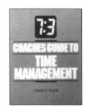

Coaches Guide to Sport Injuries

**J. David Bergeron, MEd, and
Holly Greene, PhD, ATC, RPT**

Coaches Guide
1989 • Paper • 232 pp
Item BBER0037 • ISBN 0-931250-37-4
$22.00 ($32.95 Canadian)
Study Guide
1989 • Three-Ring Notebook • 272 pp
Item ACEP0203 • ISBN 0-87322-227-X
$32.00 ($47.95 Canadian)

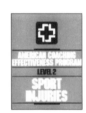

Coaches Guide to Sport Rehabilitation

Steven R. Tippett, PT, ATC

Coaches Guide
1990 • Paper • 168 pp
Item PTIP0399 • ISBN 0-88011-399-5
$22.00 ($32.95 Canadian)
Study Guide
1991 • Comb-Bound • 160 pp
Item ACEP0208 • ISBN 0-88011-447-9
$32.00 ($47.95 Canadian)

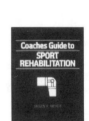

Coaches Guide to Drugs and Sport

**Kevin R. Ringhofer, PhD, and
Martha E. Harding**

1996 • Paper • 208 pp
Item PRIN0715 • ISBN 0-87322-715-8
$18.95 ($27.95 Canadian)

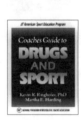

Prices are subject to change.

Human Kinetics
The Premier Publisher for Sports & Fitness
http://www.humankinetics.com

2335